So you're

Prostate
Surgery

ERIC A. KLEIN MD
LEAH JAMNICKY RN
ROBERT NAM MD

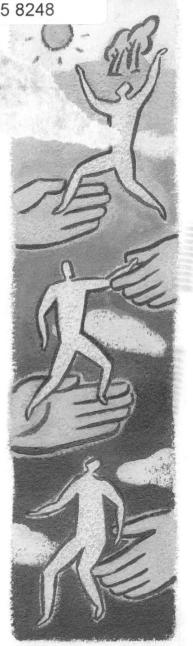

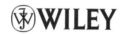WILEY

Published by John Wiley & Sons, Inc., 111 River Street, Hoboken, NJ 07030

First published in Canada in a somewhat different form by SCRIPT Medical Press, Inc. in 2003.
Copyright © 2003 SCRIPT Medical Press, Inc.

Library of Congress Cataloging-in-Publication Data

Klein, Eric A., 1955-
   So you're having prostate surgery / Eric A. Klein, Leah Jamnicky,
Robert Nam.
        p. cm.
Includes bibliographical references and index.
   ISBN 0-470-83344-0 (Paper)
   1. Prostate—Cancer—Surgery—Popular works. 2. Patient education.
I. Jamnicky, Leah. II. Nam, Robert. III. Title.
RC280.P7 K54 2003
616.99'463—dc22

                                    2003020690

General Editor and Series Creator: Helen Byrt
Editors: Dennis Jeanes, Jenny Lass
Copy Editor: Andrea Knight
Series Design: Brian Cartwright
Typesetting: Angela Bobotsis
Cover Illustration: Ross Paul Lindo
Author Photographs: Don Gerda, Cleveland Clinic Foundation; Sears Portrait Studio;
Doug Nicholson, Media Source;
Book Illustrations: Zane Waldman
Publishing Consultant: Malcolm Lester & Associates

Photograph on page 73 courtesy of Media Source.

The publisher has made every effort to obtain permissions for use of copyrighted material in this book; any errors or omissions will be corrected in the next printing.

Printed and bound in Canada
10 9 8 7 6 5 4 3 2 1

To all those patients who face the decision of "what to do?" when diagnosed with BPH or prostate cancer.

———

E.A.K.

To my loving parents, Paul and Betty, my brother, Paul, and my sisters, Lydia and Rachael, and their wonderful families.

———

L.J.

To my loving wife, Yuna, and my son, Matthew.

———

R.N.

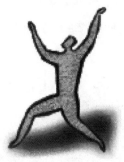

[OTHER BOOKS *in the* SERIES]

So You're Having
Heart Cath and Angioplasty

So You're Having
Heart Bypass Surgery

So You're Having A
Hysterectomy

acknowledgments

The publisher's heartfelt thanks are due to many individuals who believed in this book and worked to make it happen. Dennis Jeanes, Jenny Lass, Angela Bobotsis, Zane Waldman, Sarah Ternoway, Andrea Knight, Debra Beck, Malcolm Lester, Harold Lass, Michèle George, and Dana Habib rode the rollercoaster with a steady eye and a firm grip. The book is better because Dr. Stuart McCluskey, Lucia Evans RN, and Dr. Keyvan Karkouti spent time with it. Others who supported our authors and deserve our thanks include Dr. Andrew Matthew, Minnie Ho, Susan Anonby RN, Leah Gabriel, Judy Costello RN, Anneta Ramsamugh, Lisa Andrews RN, Chrisa Goebel RN, Rachael Brassard BSc, and Lydia Bartell RN. Finally, to the prostate surgery patients who graciously shared their experiences so that others might benefit from them: thank you.

disclaimer

THE INFORMATION PROVIDED IN THIS BOOK MAY NOT apply to all patients, all clinical situations, all hospitals, or all eventualities, and is not intended to be a substitute for the advice of a qualified physician or other medical professional. Always consult a qualified physician about anything that affects your health, especially before starting an exercise program or using a complementary therapy not prescribed by your doctor.

The publisher and the authors make no representations or warranties with respect to the accuracy or completeness of the contents of this work and specifically disclaim all warranties, including without limitation any implied warranties of fitness for a particular purpose. No warranty may be created or extended by any promotional statements. Neither the publisher nor the authors shall be liable for any damages arising herefrom.

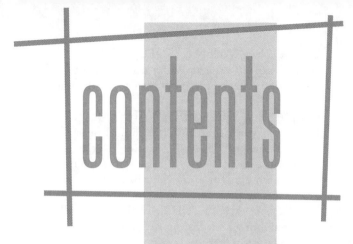
contents

INTRODUCTION ix

Chapter 1 — PROSTATE DISEASE AND YOU 1
All about the prostate ⌒ Benign prostatic hyperplasia (BPH)
⌒ Prostate cancer

Chapter 2 — TESTS AND MEASUREMENTS 13
Tests for urinary tract symptoms ⌒ Tests for prostate cancer
⌒ The PSA test ⌒ Understanding tumors

Chapter 3 — IS PROSTATE SURGERY RIGHT FOR YOU? 28
Reasons for recommending surgery ⌒ TURP ⌒ Radical
prostatectomy ⌒ Other options for BPH ⌒ Other options
for cancer ⌒ The pros and cons of watchful waiting, radiation,
medication, and surgery

Chapter 4 — GETTING READY FOR YOUR SURGERY 48
Mental preparation ⌒ Pre-surgery arrangements
⌒ The pre-admission clinic ⌒ Understanding consent
⌒ Bowel preparation ⌒ Planning for a blood transfusion

Chapter 5 — THE DAY OF YOUR SURGERY 62
What to pack for your hospital stay ⌒ Arrival at the hospital
⌒ Pre-surgery preparations ⌒ Transfer to the operating room
⌒ Advice for friends and family

Chapter 6 — THE SURGICAL PROCEDURES 69
The anesthesiologist's role ⌒ Step-by-step guide to TURP
⌒ Step-by-step guide to radical prostatectomy

Chapter 7 — WHEN IT'S ALL OVER 77
What to expect when you wake up ⌒ Your catheter and other tubes
⌒ Pain management ⌒ Activity on the ward ⌒ Going home

Chapter 8 — RECOVERING AT HOME 87
Caring for your incisions after radical prostatectomy ⌒ Managing
your catheter ⌒ Exercise, driving, work, flying, sex ⌒ Follow-up
visits ⌒ Side effects ⌒ Treatments for incontinence
⌒ Treatments for erectile dysfunction

Chapter 9 — HOW YOU CAN HELP YOURSELF 105
Understanding and dealing with emotions ⌒ Managing stress
⌒ Relaxation techniques ⌒ Exercise ⌒ BPH and diet
⌒ Prostate cancer and diet ⌒ Rediscovering sex

Chapter 10 — HAS MY SURGERY WORKED? 119
Measuring success after TURP ⌒ Measuring success after radical
prostatectomy ⌒ Additional cancer treatments

Chapter 11 — MEDICATIONS 128
Drugs for BPH ⌒ Drugs for Prostate Cancer ⌒ Drugs used before,
during, and after surgery ⌒ Side effects

Chapter 12 — FUTURE DIRECTIONS IN PROSTATE TREATMENT . .139
Clinical trials ⌒ New advances in BPH ⌒ New advances in prostate
cancer treatment

Chapter 13 — WHO'S WHO OF HOSPITAL STAFF 143

GLOSSARY 149
RESOURCES 153
YOUR DIARY 155
INDEX 162

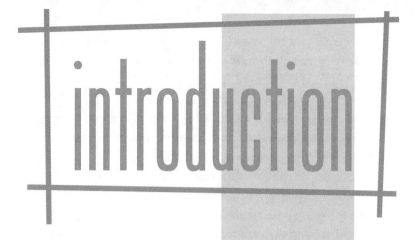

introduction

hances are, you may already be familiar with the way a walnut-sized piece of tissue located in a most intimate part of your anatomy can interfere with your life—or worse, make you terminally ill. If you or a loved one might be facing prostate surgery in the near future, we hope our book will bring you some peace of mind and help you to better understand your options so that you can make an informed treatment decision. As health professionals who are involved daily in the clinical management of prostate disease, we know from experience that the more you know about "what happens next," the easier it will be for you to decide whether surgery is right for you.

First, we'll outline conditions that affect the prostate and how they're diagnosed. We'll cover prostate anatomy and the differences between benign (non-cancerous) and malignant (cancerous) prostate disease. If you've never experienced a trans-rectal ultrasound or a prostate biopsy, we encourage you to acquaint yourself with these diagnostic procedures (outlined in Chapter 2) so that you feel prepared for the tests you may have to undergo.

We then place the pros and cons of surgery into context with other treatment options, including "watchful waiting." But if you and your physician decide that surgery is your best option, our book will give you a step-by-step description of what to expect before, during, and after your operation, including tips for more effective healing, pain management, and lifestyle changes. How you manage your recovery after prostate surgery is, as you'll discover, almost as important to your quality of life as the procedure itself.

To help you track your journey to better health, we've included a personal diary at the back of this book where you can write down your medical history, important contact information, appointment dates, medications, and symptoms.

Although the wealth of detail we've provided to you may seem a bit overwhelming, arming yourself with this information will help you to become an active participant in managing your disease, and to regain control of your long-term well-being. Above all, we encourage you to stay positive.

Good luck!

—Eric A. Klein, MD
—Leah Jamnicky, RN
—Robert Nam, MD

Chapter

prostate disease and you

What Happens in this Chapter

- Who gets prostate disease?
- Anatomy of the urinary system and prostate gland
- The facts on benign prostatic hyperplasia (BPH)
- The facts on prostate cancer

The prostate gland has several functions. As well as producing fluids that nourish sperm, it acts as a urinary sphincter and its muscles help semen flow during ejaculation. That's why the prostate is strategically located just below the bladder and surrounds the upper part of the urethra, the tube from which you urinate and ejaculate. Benign, or non-cancerous, enlargement of the prostate is prevalent among men over age 50. Prostate cancer is the commonest type of cancer in men and the second leading cause of male cancer death. Although surgery for benign prostate disease is reserved for cases that don't respond to other therapies, surgical removal of the prostate remains one of the most important and useful ways to treat cancer. Both procedures aim to restore and preserve quality of life.

The Facts About Prostate Disease

THERE ARE THREE KINDS OF PROSTATE DISORDER: INFLAMMATION of the prostate gland (**prostatitis**), benign prostate enlargement or **benign prostatic hyperplasia** (**BPH**), and prostate cancer. All three conditions are common, with prostate cancer and BPH being more common in men aged 50 and older. Although they can have the same symptoms, they all have different causes. Only prostate cancer and BPH can be treated with surgery; an inflamed prostate is usually treated with medication.

The older you get, the more likely you are to have an enlarged prostate. Only 8 percent of men aged 30 to 40 have enlarged prostates, compared to 50 percent of men aged 50 to 60, and 90 percent of men aged 80 or more.

However, an enlarged prostate is not an immediate ticket to the operating room. BPH is almost considered a normal part of aging. And it is important to remember that the condition doesn't automatically mean that you increase your risk of developing cancer. The improved treatment options available to men with BPH today mean that only about 1 in 20 patients needs surgery—those with the most severe clinical symptoms or who develop medical problems from the condition.

Even if you have prostate cancer, the good news is that this disease is being caught more frequently and earlier as a result of improved awareness and new screening procedures introduced in the late 1980s. In 1997, prostate cancer accounted for about 28 percent of all newly diagnosed cases of cancer in men—surpassing lung cancer—and is now the most common male cancer. However, with current treatment methods, most men with localized disease can be cured.

Prostate Anatomy and Function

The prostate is a good example of evolution's economy of design, making do with one set of plumbing instead of creating two. However, this piggybacking of the reproductive system onto the urinary system creates problems that most often appear at a time in a man's life when he might be happier passing urine in a strong, steady stream than passing on his DNA.

The Urinary Journey

Urine is filtered from the blood by the kidneys and then runs into the bladder through two tubes, called the **ureters** (see Figure I–I). The bladder consists of a balloon-like membrane surrounded by layers of smooth-muscle tissue, collectively called the **detrusor**. When you urinate, nerve pathways signal the detrusor to contract. After you empty your bladder, your brain signals the detrusor muscle to relax. Much of the conscious control you have over urination is from learning as a child to inhibit spontaneous contractions of your bladder.

Figure 1–1. The Urinary Journey

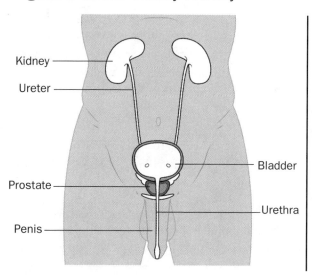

Kidney
Ureter
Bladder
Prostate
Urethra
Penis

The kidneys filter the blood and eliminate waste products as urine. The urine flows through the ureters and collects in the bladder. When you urinate, the bladder contracts to push the urine out through the urethra.

The bladder is an amazing organ that can expand to hold about half a liter (16 oz) of urine before you have a conscious sensation of fullness. You produce approximately 1.5 liters (48 oz) of urine every 24 hours. Rings of muscle (called the **internal sphincter**) at the bottom of the bladder and prostate gland form a neck that can open up or clamp shut.

Urine leaves the bladder through a tube called the **urethra** and exits through the penis. You control the flow of urine with a donut-shaped muscle called the **external sphincter**, which acts as a stop-valve when contracted.

How Do You Urinate?

When you decide to urinate, the bladder contracts, the internal sphincter of the bladder's neck relaxes and urine flows into the urethra. When you consciously relax the external sphincter, urine passes out.

The Urethra-Prostate Connection

In addition to emptying the bladder, the urethra serves as the passageway for ejaculating sperm. Thin tubes called the **vas deferens** loop back from each testicle about 46 cm (18 inches) along both sides of the bladder (see Figure 1–2). These tubes transport sperm with a rippling, muscular motion. Also entering from each side are ducts from the **seminal vesicles**, tubular structures tucked up underneath the bladder. The vas deferens and the seminal vesicles meet, then merge with the urethra.

What Is Semen? [**MORE DETAIL**]

Semen is made up of sperm and a lubricating, nourishing fluid called **seminal fluid**. Most of the seminal fluid is produced by the seminal vesicles. The rest is made by other organs, including the prostate.

Figure 1–2. The Urethra-Prostate Connection

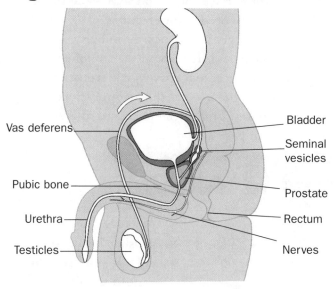

Vas deferens

Pubic bone

Urethra

Testicles

Bladder

Seminal vesicles

Prostate

Rectum

Nerves

Sperm are produced by the testes, and then travel up though the vas deferens. The sperm mix with seminal fluids from the prostate and other glands to form semen, which leaves the body through the urethra during ejaculation.

So where does the prostate fit into all of this? Although we call it the prostate "gland," the prostate is actually a collection of glands and smooth-muscle fibers encased in a fibrous, muscular capsule. The prostate sits across the upper urethra, the vas deferens, and the ducts of the seminal vesicles, between the neck of the bladder and the external sphincter.

The prostate consists of an inner zone (called the **transition zone**) and an outer (or **peripheral**) zone, and is also divided into right and left sides, called **lobes** (see Figure 1–3). Prostate cancer usually arises from the peripheral zone, whereas BPH usually originates from the transition zone. The wide portion nearest the bladder is the **base**, and the tip farthest from the bladder is the **apex**. Just a few millimeters behind the prostate is the front wall of the rectum.

Between them run networks of microscopic blood vessels and the all-important nerve pathways that are needed for erections.

At birth, the prostate is no bigger than a pea. At puberty, it grows rapidly, attaining its adult shape and size (about the size of a small walnut) at around age 20. During sexual activity, it secretes a thin, milky fluid that is pumped into the urethra through tiny ducts. Once there, it mixes with the rest of the semen to make it flow more easily (see More Detail box on page 4).

Benign Prostate Enlargement

[KEY POINT]

The symptoms of prostate enlargement are:

- a sudden, urgent need to urinate (**urgency** or **urge incontinence**)
- an increase in the number of bathroom visits during the day or night (**frequency**)
- a weak or intermittent urinary stream
- not being able to urinate at all (**urinary retention**)
- straining when urinating
- hesitation before urine flow starts
- feeling the bladder hasn't emptied completely
- dribbling or leakage
- painful urination
- occasionally, blood in the urine (**hematuria**) or urinary tract infection

At around age 50, the prostate begins to enlarge as a result of a condition called benign prostatic hyperplasia or BPH. This happens when benign clusters of cells called **adenomas** begin to form within the transition zone of the prostate (see Figure 1–4). Over time, these multiply (hyperplasia) and thus slowly increase the size of the prostate. As it enlarges, the prostate slowly compresses the urethra and urination may become difficult.

Figure 1–3. A Normal Prostate Gland

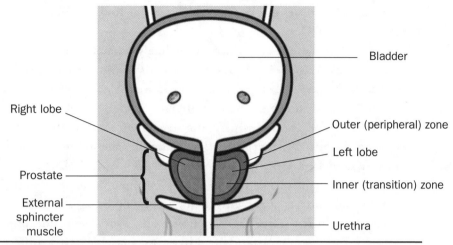

Bladder

Right lobe

Outer (peripheral) zone

Left lobe

Prostate

Inner (transition) zone

External sphincter muscle

Urethra

The prostate gland sits beneath the bladder. It consists of an inner zone and an outer zone, and is divided into right and left lobes.

Figure 1–4. Benign Prostatic Hyperplasia (BPH)

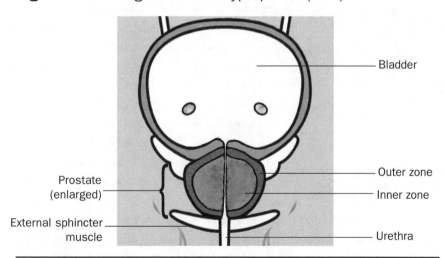

Bladder

Prostate (enlarged)

Outer zone

Inner zone

External sphincter muscle

Urethra

BPH occurs when the cells in the inner zone of the prostate start to multiply and grow. The growing prostate may compress the urethra and the bladder, making urination difficult.

Whatever the causes of prostate enlargement (see More Detail box on page 10), the condition can make passing urine (**voiding**) difficult. These difficulties are known collectively as **lower urinary tract symptoms** (**LUTS**).

If you are having trouble voiding, it is likely because your urethra and bladder neck are being squeezed, or constricted. In BPH, this constriction happens very gradually, so you might not realize it at first. See if this scenario sounds familiar:

One day, you notice that your urine stream isn't as forceful as it used to be. Eventually, there's a delay in starting the urine flow, and no matter how hard you try, the flow tapers off to a dribbling conclusion. Or perhaps you experience the phenomenon captured by the apt French phrase *pis en deux*, which describes passing a second large volume of urine after the first flow stops. Worst of all, despite your best efforts, you constantly feel like your bladder hasn't quite emptied.

More annoying still are the storage symptoms that develop as a result of the hard work your bladder has to do to overcome the voiding problems. The strain of not being able to fully empty your bladder makes you go to the bathroom urgently and more frequently. After you relieve yourself, your bladder still feels partly full. The bladder's signals to urinate are so strong that you are repeatedly woken up during the night, a condition called **nocturia**. Recognize the pattern? For most men, this is an all-too-familiar description of how BPH encroaches on their quality of life.

> "I had started to wake up in the middle of the night and had trouble urinating sometimes. It took a lot of coercing to get a stream going."
>
> **Ray**

BPH can cause other problems. Urine that has been sitting in the bladder for a long time can become a breeding ground for common bacteria, and cause infections of the bladder and urinary tract. One sign of an infection is a burning sensation when urinating. If you've been diagnosed with BPH, and have been experiencing repeated bladder and urinary tract infections, surgery may be a better option than recurring bouts of illness and prescriptions for antibiotics (see Chapter 3). This "old" urine can also form crystals that then grow into stones. Passing a stone through the urethra is an experience few men forget and could lead to the need for surgery. However, passing these kinds of stones is rare, and is usually accompanied by an infection and hematuria.

Another symptom of BPH is **acute urinary retention**, with which you suddenly lose the ability to urinate. The bladder fills up and becomes extremely painful. The trigger for acute urinary retention can be as simple as standing in the cold with an overly full bladder, prolonged bed rest, or constipation. A minor infection may also cause the urethra to swell or the prostate to enlarge just enough to complete the blockage. The most effective immediate treatment for this urgent complication is for a doctor to insert a **catheter** (a thin, hollow tube) into the bladder to drain the urine.

Occasionally, as a result of weak signals between the spinal cord and bladder, urine retention can become chronic. A man's bladder can fill up painlessly over a period of months (even years!) until it expands to many times its normal size. He may experience vague abdominal and pelvic discomfort, and can only pass urine in small quantities. Every once in a while there may be leakage, but generally the man is unaware that his bladder is overly full. Very rarely, the pressure from the bladder can rise to such an extent that urine is forced back along the ureters to the kidneys, causing harm. Once again, catheterization is the immediate first step to recovery, usually followed by surgery. However, a severely enlarged or distended bladder may never return to its normal size and the stretched detrusor will have trouble contracting and emptying the bladder properly.

Prostate Cancer

Compared to other forms of cancer, prostate tumors are slow growing. A tumor that is confined within the prostate gland may take 5

New Theories for an Old Problem

There are a number of theories about why prostate enlargement happens. The most popular theory blames the principal male hormone **testosterone**. After puberty and well into old age, the prostate is routinely bathed with testosterone. Once inside the prostate, testosterone is converted into an even more powerful hormone, **dihydrotestosterone** (**DHT**), which stimulates the prostate's glandular cells to grow during puberty. Not surprisingly, DHT is the chief suspect in mid- and late-life prostatic glandular enlargement.

However, some experts place the blame on DHT's female counterpart, **estrogen**, which is normally present at low levels in men. The relative proportion of estrogen increases as men age and produce less testosterone. This change in hormonal proportions could possibly trigger prostate enlargement.

The "late bloomers" theory argues that certain types of prostate cells only become active later in life, when they become sensitive to DHT and other growth signals. Another theory claims that some of the glandular cells might not know when to call it quits, disobeying normal self-destruct orders and multiplying instead.

Whatever the exact mechanism, genetics may help to explain why some men develop BPH and others don't. Studies have shown that men who need surgery for enlarged prostates often have a family history—that is, they have a father or brother with the same problem. However, a "BPH gene" has not yet been identified.

Figure 1–5. Prostate Cancer

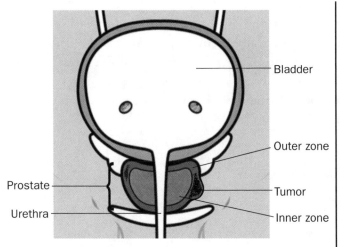

Bladder

Outer zone

Prostate

Tumor

Urethra

Inner zone

There are usually few symptoms in the early stages of prostate cancer because the tumor tends to grow slowly in the outer zone of the prostate, away from the urethra. In later stages, the tumor may grow large enough to squeeze the urethra or other structures.

to 15 years to spread to other organs. Therefore, the younger you are, the more likely it is that you'll be a candidate for surgery or radiation therapy before the cancer has had time to spread. If you are older and have no symptoms, watchful waiting may be an option (see pages 36–37).

Early stage prostate cancer generally doesn't cause noticeable symptoms because it occurs in the outer layer of the prostate gland and does not interfere with urination (see Figure 1–5). PSA testing (see pages 17–19) means that most prostate cancers are now detected in the early stages.

When the tumor has increased in size it can cause symptoms similar to BPH. Back pain and bone pain may mean that the cancer has spread to other parts of the body, such as the spine and pelvis.

"I guess the hardest part was accepting the fact that I did have prostate cancer. I was 57, I was running 3 or 4 miles every day, I was playing tennis 3 or 4 times a week, I was about 20 pounds lighter than I am now. And it was inconceivable to me that I could have anything wrong with me."

Nat

What Happens Next?

Depending on your situation, your doctor will order tests to confirm benign prostate enlargement or prostate cancer, and rule out other possible causes for your symptoms. Early detection of prostate cancer is always an advantage because it is easier to cure at this early stage, with one of the many available treatment options.

Chapter 2

tests and measurements

What Happens in this Chapter

- Tests for urinary tract symptoms
- Tests for prostate cancer
- Interpreting your PSA
- Understanding tumors

There are several tests available for detecting benign prostatic hyperplasia and prostate cancer, and finding out what is causing your symptoms. It's an anxious but constructive time because you're taking the first step toward getting some answers and ultimately feeling better.

Tests for Lower Urinary Tract Symptoms (LUTS)

THERE IS A SPECIFIC GROUP OF TESTS THAT YOUR DOCTOR WILL want you to undergo if you start experiencing LUTS. While some of them might be uncomfortable, they can tell your physician a lot about what the problem is and how best to help you.

AUA Symptom Score

Along with a physical examination, your answers to this questionnaire, designed by the American Urological Association, will help your physician gain a more accurate understanding of the nature and severity of your urinary symptoms (see More Detail box on page 15). The **AUA symptom score** is particularly helpful in diagnosing BPH and deciding whether treatment is a good idea. It is also helpful in monitoring how well you respond to treatment.

Uroflow

During your assessment, the doctor may send you for a **uroflow test**. This machine measures how fast and how well you can empty your bladder.

Abdominal Ultrasound

This imaging tool is used to see inside the kidneys and bladder. Ultrasound works on the same principle as marine SONAR: sound waves are emitted and allowed to bounce off objects in their path. The echoes created from the bounced waves produce an image of what the ultrasound signal bumped into. The ultrasound probe works at very high frequencies (well beyond human hearing) to provide fine detail at a range of several centimeters. The image that the ultrasound test produces can reveal stones, and other problems with

The AUA Symptom Index

Date:	Not at all	Less than 1 time in 5	Less than half the time	About half the time	More than half the time	Almost always
Circle Your Score for Each Below						
1. Over the past month or so, how often have you had the sensation of not emptying your bladder completely after you finished urinating?	0	1	2	3	4	5
2. Over the past month or so, how often have you had to urinate again less than two hours after you finished urinating?	0	1	2	3	4	5
3. Over the past month or so, how often have you found that you stopped and started again several times when you urinated?	0	1	2	3	4	5
4. Over the past month or so, how often have you found it difficult to postpone urination?	0	1	2	3	4	5
5. Over the past month or so, how often have you had a weak urinary stream?	0	1	2	3	4	5
6. Over the past month or so, how often have you had to push or strain to begin urination?	0	1	2	3	4	5
7. Over the last month, how many times did you most typically get up to urinate from the time you went to bed at night until the time you got up in the morning?	0	1	2	3	4	5

Total symptom score =
Sum of questions 1 to 7 = [   ] /35
Discuss this score with your doctor

Source: Barry MJ, et al. *The Journal of Urology* 1992.

the kidneys, ureters, or bladder. This test is often used to rule out other possible reasons for urinary tract symptoms. It has no side effects and is non-invasive, which means that no equipment will penetrate your outer layer of skin.

Cystoscopy

A **cytoscope** is a slender, flexible, fiber-optic device that is passed down your urethra, through the prostate, and into your bladder. It allows your urologist to look directly at your urinary tract. The reason for doing cytoscopy is to rule out other causes for your symptoms. Cytoscopy can identify abnormalities in your bladder and prostate gland that other tests may not be able to reveal, such as **urethral stricture** (narrowing of the urethra) or **bladder stones**, which can mimic the symptoms of prostate enlargement. It also helps your urologist map out your specific anatomy for any future surgical treatments that may be required.

Your urethra will be numbed with an anesthetic gel before the cytoscope is inserted. For the first 24 hours after cystoscopy you may experience minor irritation or bleeding when you urinate.

Tests for Prostate Cancer

Digital Rectal Exam (DRE)

Touch tells a lot, which is why a **digital rectal exam** as part of an annual physical examination is recommended for all men over age 50. If you are at higher risk of having prostate cancer—for example, if you have a family history of prostate cancer or you are African American—it is advisable that you start having regular DRE tests (and PSA tests—see pages 17-19) at age 40. The exact age at which you should start having regular tests depends on how many of your family members are affected with prostate cancer, and you should discuss this with your physician.

For a DRE, the physician inserts a gloved, lubricated finger into the patient's rectum and feels the prostate for size, tenderness, and nodules. When a prostate is enlarged, it often loses the central groove that separates its left and right lobes. Occasionally, the physician may feel a tumor on the prostate's surface as a hard, distinct lump.

Although DREs are useful, touch has its limits. With the widespread use of PSA testing (see below), most prostate cancer is now detected in the early stages, before it can be felt on a DRE. It is also possible to have urinary tract symptoms due to enlargement of the part of the prostate that surrounds the urethra even if it does not feel very enlarged on a DRE. The true value of a DRE comes from annual repetition as part of a general physical exam, so that your doctor has a baseline—a sense of what's normal for your body—from which to gauge possible changes.

PSA Test

Until the late 1980s, a digital rectal exam was the only way to detect prostate disease early. Now annual screening and diagnostic procedures usually involve a PSA blood test. **Prostate specific antigen (PSA)** is a protein produced by the prostate that helps keep semen in liquid form. Prostate cancer cells produce more PSA than healthy cells, so this test is considered a reasonably reliable gauge for detecting early disease.

The amount of PSA is measured in **nanograms** (ng)—an unimaginably tiny billionth of a gram!—per milliliter (mL) of blood. A level below 4 ng/mL is considered to be normal. However, this is just a reference level, and the significance of each patient's PSA level will be assessed on an individual basis. Many factors can raise PSA levels apart from cancer, including normal growth of the prostate gland as you age (see More Detail box on page 18), so if you

A PSA test is a useful alert for prostate cancer, but like all tests, it has limitations. It can give a false positive because other factors apart from cancer can cause high PSA levels. In BPH, which occurs naturally as you age, there are more cells producing PSA, which can raise blood levels of PSA. If the prostate becomes inflamed (a condition called prostatitis), more PSA leaks into the bloodstream through the damaged lining of the gland, resulting in quite high PSA levels. Recent ejaculation or a biopsy can also artificially raise PSA levels. By contrast, PSA levels can be artificially lowered by certain medications (finasteride and dutasteride) (see page 136).

PSA Level (ng/mL)	Likelihood of Prostate Cancer
2.5 to 4.0	20% to 25%
4.0 to 10.0	30% to 50%
Greater than 10.0	Approximately 70%

Scientists are constantly working to develop better PSA tests. For example, one approach focuses on the amount of free PSA—PSA not bound to protein—in the blood. Free PSA testing appears to be significantly more accurate at detecting cancer in some patients with particular PSA values, such as the 4 to 10 ng/mL range, and can eliminate the need for some prostate biopsies.

The rate of change of PSA over time (called PSA velocity or PSAV) can also be a more accurate indication of whether you have cancer. One important study found that if your PSA levels increase by 0.75 ng/mL per year or more, your chances of having prostate cancer are high.

have a level slightly above 4 ng/mL your physician may consider this to be normal for you, and take no further action. On the other hand, if your PSA is just below 4 ng/mL but you have no obvious explanation for a raised PSA level, your physician may be concerned about it. The reason for this is that studies have shown that men with PSAs between 2.5 and 4.0 ng/mL have a 20 to 25 percent chance of having prostate cancer.

In general, however, if any abnormal PSA value is found your doctor should repeat the PSA test, and he or she may also suggest a prostate biopsy.

Prostate Biopsy

The only way to determine whether you have prostate cancer or not is to perform a prostate biopsy. This procedure involves using a needle to obtain a small piece of prostate tissue, which is then processed and examined under a microscope by another doctor, called a **pathologist**, to identify any prostate cancer cells.

Ultrasound is used during the prostate biopsy to create an image of the prostate and help the physician guide the biopsy needle into the prostate gland. The ultrasound probe and biopsy device are inserted into your rectum, so the procedure is called **transrectal ultrasound-guided biopsy (TRUS)**. The ultrasound image will also allow your physician to assess the size of your prostate gland and see any obvious tumors,

"My doctor said, 'Your PSA has gone up to 4 and I think you should see a urologist again.' And I didn't know much about my body. Had I known a bit more about my body I would have insisted on many things prior to that, but I didn't. And that's my goal now, to try and get men to find out a bit about their bodies...If I had known that it was rising for a reason I would have insisted on a biopsy."

Ray

although in most cases the tumors are microscopic and cannot be seen. For this reason, your physician will take several biopsies randomly throughout the gland to increase the chances of detecting any cancer tissue.

With the ultrasound probe to guide his or her actions from a monitor, the physician uses the probe's spring-loaded hollow needles to quickly pierce the rectal wall, enter the prostate, and retrieve multiple cylinders of tissue 1.5 mm (1/32 inch) in diameter. The exact number of samples taken will depend on your own situation, but in general, expect about 8 to 12 passes. Don't worry—you will be given a local anesthetic to numb the area first. The samples are then sent to a pathology lab for analysis. The whole procedure takes about 15 to 20 minutes.

[**KEY POINT**]

About 10 days before your biopsy, you will need to stop taking ASA (e.g., Aspirin), other pain relief (such as ibuprofen), blood-thinning medication (such as Coumadin), or vitamin E because these may make you bleed more heavily afterward. You should also tell your physician if you have problems with your heart valves or have prosthetics that require antibiotics before any type of medical or dental procedures. In this case, you will need to take additional antibiotics before your biopsy.

Preparing for a Biopsy

A TRUS-guided biopsy has a few more risks than other tests you'll undergo because it's more invasive. Rest assured that every precaution is taken to minimize your discomfort and risk of infection. The night before the biopsy, you may be asked to give yourself an enema or take a laxative to clean out your lower bowels, which will help make the biopsy site clean. In addition, you'll be prescribed an antibiotic that should be taken before and after the biopsy until the course of medication is complete.

After the Biopsy

After the procedure, you may experience bleeding from your rectum or penis and there may be blood in your stool, urine, or semen. This can last for up to 2 weeks or more. Don't be alarmed by this, it is quite normal.

Some men feel a little discomfort in the prostate following the procedure, when the local anesthetic wears off, so you may want to have the option of taking the day off work. However, most men are able to leave the hospital on their own without any difficulty and return to work right away. Pain relief such as acetaminophen (e.g., Tylenol) will quickly relieve some of the bruised, achy feeling.

Repeat Biopsies

Sometimes, a repeat biopsy is recommended, even if the first results are negative for cancer. There are several reasons your physician might want you to undergo additional biopsies. Because less than 1 percent of the total prostate gland is sampled, the first biopsy could miss the prostate cancer in the gland. Indeed, it has been found that 15 to 30 percent of prostate cancer can be detected from a repeat biopsy after the first biopsy came out negative.

Another reason for doing a second biopsy is that non-cancerous but abnormal cells might be found in the first biopsy. Men with these non-cancerous conditions, known as **prostatic intraepithelial neoplasia (PIN)** or **atypical small acinar cell proliferation (ASAP)**, have a 1 in 2 risk of having or developing prostate cancer, so a repeat biopsy is essential.

Some specialists favor a procedure called **saturation biopsy**, in which you go to sleep under a general anesthetic and a larger number of samples are taken. This can be helpful in finding prostate cancer in cases where multiple biopsies have shown no evidence of cancer. You and your urologist will need to decide if this option is right for you.

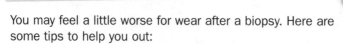

Taking Control After a Biopsy

You may feel a little worse for wear after a biopsy. Here are some tips to help you out:

- Have the option of taking the rest of the day off work
- Take along a trusted companion to help you get home afterward
- Drink fluids, but NOT alcohol
- Wait at 24 to 48 hours before having sex or doing any strenuous activity
- Contact your doctor if after 24 hours you experience fever, chills, difficulty passing urine, or excessive bleeding.

Understanding Tumors

Your biopsy results are usually available within 7 days, depending on the hospital. A pathologist who specializes in interpreting cellular anatomy will examine your tissue samples and let your physician know whether or not you have cancer. If the pathologist finds evidence of cancer, he or she can also determine how aggressive the cancer appears to be.

How Aggressive Is Your Cancer?

In simple terms, an "aggressive" cancer is one that is likely to spread rapidly to other parts of your body, such as the bones. To decide how aggressive a case of prostate cancer is, physicians use a grading system called the **Gleason score**. The pathologist who examines your tumor cells will assign the Gleason score—usually a number between 2 and 10. Patients with a Gleason score of 10 have a very aggressive-appearing prostate cancer, while the cancer in patients with a Gleason score of 2 to 5 appears very benign. The higher the score, the greater is the chance that the cancer has already spread (see More Detail box below) or will come back after surgery or radiation.

Your Gleason Score **[MORE DETAIL]**

If you have prostate cancer, your Gleason score—based on the appearance of your cancer cells under a microscope—will help your physician decide how aggressive your cancer is and what treatment you need.

Gleason Score	Percentage of Men with Prostate Cancer	What This Means
2 to 5	10 percent	Rarely spreads outside the prostate and no treatment may be necessary apart from regular follow-up.
6 to 7	80 percent	Likely to spread; usually requires treatment with surgery or radiation, depending on one's age and general health.
8 to 10	10 percent	Very likely to spread; aggressive treatment needed, with surgery, radiation, or hormones.

The other factor that your physician considers is your PSA level. As is the case with the Gleason score, patients with a higher PSA level have more aggressive cancer. Patients with a PSA of 20 ng/mL or more have a poorer prognosis than patients with levels lower than 20 ng/mL.

Has Your Cancer Spread?

Your treatment will also depend on the **stage** of your prostate cancer, i.e., whether it has already spread outside of your prostate gland. Prostate cancer can spread to areas immediately beside the gland, to lymph nodes, to your bones, or to other organs.

The most common way that physicians stage prostate cancer is the **TNM staging system** (see More Detail box on page 25). TNM stands for the three stages that cancer moves through as it spreads: "T" for tumor, "N" for (lymph) nodes, and "M" for **metastases** (cancer growths in bones and other organs).

The "T" is usually assessed by a digital rectal exam by your physician. The "N" and "M" components need to be assessed by X-ray tests such as a **CAT scan** (see page 26). You may not need these additional tests if your cancer has a low risk of spreading—that is, if you have both a low Gleason score and a low PSA level. The decision as to whether further staging tests are needed will be made by your oncologist, based on the look of your own tumor.

If your cancer has spread beyond the prostate gland, or **metastasized**, then removal of your prostate gland (**radical prostatectomy**) will not be a useful treatment strategy. Other treatments, such as radiation and hormonal medications, are available in this case, and do provide good cancer control.

If your cancer is still confined to the prostate gland, you may be eligible for radical prostatectomy and your urologist will discuss this with you.

TNM Staging System

[**MORE DETAIL**]

This system helps describe the stage of development of your cancer.

Stage	Description
T1	The tumor cannot be felt or seen using ultrasound.
T1a	Cancer cells are incidentally found in 5 percent or less of tissue samples from prostate surgery for benign disease.
T1b	Cancer cells are found in more than 5 percent of surgery-sample tissue.
T1c	Cancer cells are identified by needle biopsy because of high PSA.
T2	The cancer is confined to the prostate, but can be felt as a small, well-defined nodule.
T2a	Tumors are in half a prostate lobe.
T2b	Tumors are in more than half a prostate lobe.
T2c	Tumors are in both lobes.
T3	Tumor extends through the prostate capsule.
T4	Tumor is fixed to or invades adjacent structures.
N0	Regional lymph nodes are still cancer-free.
N1	A small tumor is in a single pelvic lymph node.
N2	A medium-sized tumor is in one lymph node, or small tumors are in several nodes.
N3	A large tumor is in one or more lymph nodes.
M0	Cancer has not spread beyond the regional lymph nodes.
M1	Cancer has spread to lymph nodes distant from the regional nodes.
M1b	Cancer has invaded the bones.
M1c	Cancer has spread to other sites.

Finding Tumors Outside the Prostate

If your physician is concerned that the cancer may have spread, he or she can send you for a number of high-tech tests to confirm this. Most results take between 1 and 3 weeks, although X-ray results are available within 48 to 72 hours. If they show that the cancer has spread, your physician will be able to adjust your treatment accordingly (see Chapter 3).

Computerized Axial Tomography (CAT) Scans

Typically, CAT scans are used to try to detect whether cancer has spread from the prostate to nearby clusters of lymph nodes. Instead of a tube being placed in you, this time it's the other way around. During this test, you lie on your back inside a long rotating tube that takes narrow-beam, 360-degree, thinly layered, X-ray pictures of your body. A high-speed computer stacks each image slice one on top of the other, like a deck of cards, and produces a 3-dimensional image of your abdomen.

Before the CAT scan, you may receive an injection of special dye to heighten the contrast and thus improve the image quality of your veins, arteries, kidneys, liver, and spleen. The injection may cause a feeling of spreading warmth and, possibly, itching as it circulates throughout your body. If you have allergies, inform the radiotherapist before the procedure since it may be safer to avoid the dye. After the test, increase your intake of fluids to flush out your system. Water and juice are preferable to alcohol.

Magnetic Resonance Imaging (MRI)

This device measures the amount of magnetic energy given off by various cells. The MRI combines an extremely powerful magnet with radio waves to create high-quality images. People who have metallic implants, such as joint replacement implants, orthopedic rods and nails for fracture repair, or a pacemaker cannot undergo this test. Also, people who can't tolerate lying motionless in an enclosed tube for the length of the procedure, which may take from 20 minutes to an hour, will not be able to have an MRI. All patients fill out an in-depth questionnaire before their MRI to bring these issues to light.

Bone Scan

The purpose of this scan is to see whether your prostate cancer has spread to your bones. A small amount of **radioisotope** is injected into your bloodstream while you're lying on your back. The radioactive solution is attracted to areas of your skeleton where changes have taken place, such as fractures, infections, arthritis, or other bone diseases. A device is then passed over your body to measure the tiny amount of radioactivity the isotopes emit. If the cancer has spread to nearby bone, then it will appear as a "hot spot" since the isotope concentrates in these areas. The test has no unwanted after-effects; the amount of radioactivity involved is safe and doesn't raise your risk of developing other types of cancer.

What Happens Next?

Now that you and your physician have a clearer understanding of your condition, you can work together to take control of your health. You must decide what course of treatment is best for you and the next chapter can help you make up your mind.

Chapter 3

is prostate surgery right for you?

What Happens in this Chapter

- Reasons for recommending surgery
- The inside story on TURP for BPH
- Pros and cons of other BPH options
- The inside story on prostate cancer surgery
- Pros and cons of other cancer options

Whether you have benign prostate enlargement or prostate cancer, your medical history, physical examinations, lab tests, and imaging technologies are guides that help your physician recommend which treatments he or she thinks are best for you. However, the decision to proceed with treatment is yours. In some cases, test results are indisputable, the diagnosis certain, and the benefits of treatment obvious. But sometimes things aren't so clear-cut. Understanding the benefits and drawbacks of your options may help you make this important decision.

Benign Prostatic Hyperplasia

IF YOU HAVE BPH, THERE ARE THREE TREATMENT OPTIONS TO consider: watchful waiting, medication, and surgery. The pros and cons of these options are summarized in the chart on page 35. Most commonly, physicians tend to start with the least invasive options. Surgery is usually reserved for men whose symptoms do not improve with medication, or when BPH starts to cause serious medical problems.

BPH: The Case for Watchful Waiting

Watchful waiting is the medical term for a "wait-and-see" approach. You and your physician will keep a close eye on your symptoms, but do nothing unless something changes.

Large clinical studies indicate that BPH symptoms improve or disappear on their own in 20 to 50 percent of cases approximately. Therefore, many men do not need any treatment. However, about a third of those who choose to wait and see will experience progressive worsening of their symptoms and some may eventually lose the ability to empty their bladder. The 10-year risk for developing acute urinary retention (see page 9) is about 13 percent—or odds of slightly better than 1 in 10. The risk for requiring surgery for BPH is about 5 percent (or odds of 1 in 20). These low probabilities make watchful waiting quite attractive, especially when BPH symptoms are mild and not too bothersome.

Living with Mild Prostate Enlargement

Most men adjust to mild urinary symptoms—a visit to the washroom before leaving home, scouting out the public lavatory at the mall, taking the aisle seat at the movies, and reducing fluid intake after dinner or before bedtime.

Certain medications can aggravate BPH symptoms. If you have allergies or catch a cold, you'll have to think twice about taking

How to Decide?

- In general, start with the less invasive treatments.

- Your own health condition may mean that one or more of the alternatives is not available to you.

- If in doubt, get a second (or third) opinion from another physician. Tell them you are seeking another opinion. This is normal. Your family doctor or friends will be able to suggest alternate names.

- As with all illnesses, your condition can change over time and you may need to revise your decision.

- You are entitled to change your mind if you feel that you have made a wrong choice.

non-prescription medications known as **adrenergics** because they mimic the effects of **adrenaline** (also called **epinephrine**). This is the "fight-or-flight" hormone that evolved in mammals to speed up the body for coping with such emergencies as outrunning a lion or avoiding an oncoming car. Many decongestants contain a synthetic version of adrenaline, called **pseudoephedrine**, which relaxes the lung's bronchial passages, stimulates the heart rate, and constricts blood vessels. Another problem with adrenergics is that they constrict muscles in the prostate and bladder making it harder to urinate. Antihistamines, such as diphenhydramine (Benadryl), can also slow urine flow in some men.

Anyone who has BPH and **hypertension** (high blood pressure) or **congestive heart disease**, and is taking **diuretics**, such as chlorthalidone or hydrochlorothiazide, should discuss the risks and benefits of this drug regimen with his doctor. Diuretics (also called "water pills") decrease the amount of fluid in your body by encouraging the kidneys to produce large quantities of urine. This might be a good thing for hypertension, but clearly there's a conflict for someone who has lower urinary tract symptoms or is prone to urinary retention. However, no one should stop taking diuretics without medical supervision since these drugs are an important treatment for cardiovascular disease.

"I encourage men to enhance their knowledge base, to educate themselves so that they understand some of the "techy" terms like PSA and digital rectal exam—and that they understand the results that come from the tests."

Ron

BPH: The Case for Drug Therapy

Medication has become a popular treatment choice for BPH. In the United States, the number of prescriptions written monthly for BPH drugs increased from less than 400,000 to more than one million between 1993 and 1996. The obvious advantage of drug therapy is that it provides effective relief of BPH symptoms without surgery.

Two classes of prescription medications are used: **alpha blockers** and **5-alpha-reductase inhibitors**. For a more detailed discussion of the medications used to treat BPH, see Chapter 11. Saw palmetto, an over-the-counter herbal medication, may also help alleviate some of the mild symptoms of BPH (seee page 113).

So if these medications are effective, why does anyone opt for surgery? For one thing, although alpha blockers and 5-alpha-reductase inhibitors can slow up the progression of the disease, either alone or in combination, studies show that this does not work for all men. Symptoms can worsen during drug treatment and the risk of developing acute urinary retention still exists. Symptoms return soon after you stop taking the drugs, so you may need to take medication for the rest of your life. Also, some of the drugs aren't currently covered by public or private drug plans, so this approach may prove to be expensive. Some men also find side effects, such as dizziness, ejaculatory problems, or nasal congestion, troublesome. Although drug therapy alone can be an effective method of treating BPH, regular check-ups with your doctor are a must if this is the route you choose.

BPH: The Case for Surgery

Surgery for BPH is considered "elective"—that is, it's your choice if and when you have the procedure. For many men, their choice depends on how well they can put up with reduced urinary flow and frequent urination (especially during the night). Some can tolerate urinary tract symptoms with little difficulty; others cannot. However, you may not really have a choice under certain circumstances, such as if you experience a decline in kidney function, repeated episodes of blood in your urine, multiple urinary tract infections, and bladder stones. Surgery is also a good option if you develop **diverticulae**, abnormal pockets of tissue in the bladder that can trap urine and cause infection.

The Advantages of TURP

The surgical gold standard for treating BPH is **transurethral resection of the prostate (TURP)**. This procedure involves removing the prostate tissue that surrounds the urethra to relieve the pressure. TURP is described in detail in Chapter 6.

Studies have repeatedly shown that, after TURP, patients don't have to urinate as often and their urinary flow is much stronger.

The benefits of TURP are long-lasting, and the procedure reduces the chance that you'll need additional drug therapy. There's only a 1 in 20 chance that you'll need repeat surgery after 5 years. Repeat surgery becomes necessary if prostate tissue re-grows and obstructs the urinary passage, but this second procedure poses no greater risk than the original operation.

Recovery from TURP is fast because the procedure is done via the urethra, with no surgical incision. Once the catheter that was inserted in the urethra is removed after surgery, you should be able to urinate right away and will notice an immediate improvement in symptoms. You should be able to return to normal daily activities (light duties only) in as little as 1 week after the procedure, although complete healing usually takes about 6 weeks. TURP also generally causes few complications. Severe complications are extremely rare.

The Downsides of TURP

Although most patients do well after TURP, a few suffer a complication called **urinary retention**, in which they are unable to empty their bladder. A variety of factors contribute to this complication, such as an individual's overall health, whether he experienced acute urinary retention before the operation, and inflammation and bleeding caused by the surgery. If this happens to you, a catheter will be inserted into your bladder and removed several days later when you have healed properly. If there is excessive bleeding, the catheter will need to be irrigated with fluid in order to flush out any blood clots that may have formed.

If urinary retention occurs on a regular basis, a technique called **intermittent self-catheterization** (ISC) may help. The patient is taught to insert a catheter himself whenever urinary retention occurs, to relieve himself. For most men, this solution is only necessary for a short period and the bladder settles down in time. For a rare few, ISC may be needed indefinitely.

Another downside of TURP is that it can cause at least temporary sexual dysfunction (erection difficulties) in about 1 in 25 patients. It can also cause urinary leakage, or incontinence, in up to 1 in 100 patients. About 75 percent of patients will experience **retrograde ejaculation**, a harmless condition in which some (or all) of the ejaculate goes into the bladder, rather than out of the penis, during orgasm.

Minimally Invasive Treatments

Over the years the search has been on to find alternatives to TURP. Several minimally invasive procedures have been developed, some of which are still experimental and others are available only at some hospitals or at private clinics. They include techniques to shrink or destroy the prostate tissue (**high-intensity ultrasound, laser treatment, transurethral electrovaporization, transurethral needle ablation, hyperthermia** or **thermotherapy**) and procedures to stretch and "prop open" the urethra (**transurethral balloon dilation** and **intraurethral stents**).

Two techniques that have gained popularity more rapidly than the others are **transurethral microwave thermotherapy** (**TUMT**) and **needle ablation** (**TUNA**).

TUMT and TUNA can be performed as day procedures in a hospital or private clinic. TUMT uses microwaves to destroy the prostate tissue that is causing obstruction, while TUNA uses radiowaves to coagulate or "melt" the tissue. Although these techniques have not been studied very extensively as yet, and their long-term benefits are still unknown, they do appear to genuinely improve symptoms. The downside of these procedures is that they may not be covered by health care plans, in which case you may be in for a bill of several thousand dollars.

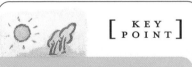

[**KEY POINT**]

Deciding to treat BPH depends primarily on how bothered you are by your urinary symptoms. Before you decide on surgery or medications, be sure to thoroughly discuss the risks and benefits of each with your urologist.

BPH Treatment—Pros and Cons

There are many factors to consider when you're deciding what treatment is best for you. This quick reference chart may help.

	Advantages	Disadvantages
Watchful Waiting	• no invasive procedures • no drugs • up to half of BPH cases resolve by themselves • reserved for mild symptoms and low risk of urinary retention	• a third of men experience progressive worsening of symptoms • must avoid over-the-counter cold remedies • water pills for hypertension worsen symptoms • silent disease progression: stones, infections, bleeding, impaired kidney function • 1 in 10 odds of acute urinary retention • 1 in 20 odds of surgery
Medications	• safe and effective way to relax prostate sphincter muscle • less urinary frequency and urgency	• benefits are dependent on drug • drugs may be required for a long time and some drugs are costly • risk of side effects • risk of urinary retention still exists
TURP	• significantly less urinary frequency and urgency • benefits long-lasting • no drugs • low risk of repeat surgery • quick recovery from a one-time event	• discomfort, hospital stay, anesthetics • rarely, acute urinary retention after surgery requiring long-term catheterization • erectile dysfunction in 1 in 25 (temporary in most cases) • incontinence in 1 in 100 • retrograde ejaculation is common

Prostate Cancer

For prostate cancer, there are currently four main options: a wait-and-see approach (watchful waiting), radiation therapy, medication, and surgical removal of the prostate (radical prostatectomy). These options are summarized on page 46. Your age, lifestyle, PSA level, and biopsy results will largely shape your options. If your physician recommends active treatment, it is worth realizing that radiation and surgery appear to be equally effective. As long as the cancer is confined to the prostate, the chances of a complete cure with either treatment are extremely good.

Prostate Cancer: The Case for Watchful Waiting

Watchful waiting involves having no treatment for your prostate cancer until you start experiencing symptoms, at which time your physician will treat the symptoms only, usually with medication.

Watchful waiting can be very appealing to men who don't want any type of treatment for prostate cancer. Unlike some other kinds of cancer, prostate cancer can be very slow growing, taking 5 to 15 years to spread and become potentially lethal. That's why many men who develop prostate cancer late in life die *with* the disease rather than *from* it.

Despite the appeal of

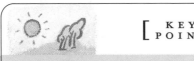

[**KEY POINT**]

Watchful waiting is not a treatment. It means doing nothing to "cure" your cancer and simply treating symptoms as they arise. If you opt for watchful waiting and your cancer spreads, your chances of a cure are greatly reduced. Your oncologist will discuss the pros and cons of watchful waiting with you, based on the characteristics of your own tumor.

"doing nothing," watchful waiting is really only an option for a select group of men. Men in their late 60s or older whose cancer appears less aggressive and men who are too ill from other causes to undergo treatment are the best candidates for watchful waiting. If your cancer has already started progressing, you will be advised to start curative treatment without delay, i.e., radiotherapy or surgery.

If you opt for waiting, you'll need to have regular check-ups. Your oncologist will do regular PSA measurements and DRE checks to determine the status of your prostate cancer.

Deciding When to Treat

For most men, particularly younger men with localized cancer, the treatment decision hinges on factors such as TMN stage, Gleason grade, and PSA level (see Chapter 2). With these factors in mind, you and your oncologist will first discuss whether treatment for your prostate cancer is necessary, and then which treatment is best for you.

> "I had come from the school where the doctor kind of recommends to you what to do. But in prostate cancer you have to make the decision for yourself. It's not made for you. You have to decide on treatment based on your own lifestyle and what you can live with down the road."
>
> Jim

Prostate Cancer: The Case for Radiation

Radiation therapy for prostate cancer has been around for many years and studies so far show that it is as effective as surgery in controlling cancer in certain kinds of patients (see More Detail box on page 38).

The two kinds of radiation treatment commonly used to treat prostate cancer are **external beam radiotherapy** and **brachytherapy**.

There are a number of factors to consider when you're trying to decide if radiation treatment is right for you. Its main advantage is that you are spared a major, invasive procedure. External beam radiotherapy does not require any anesthetic and, although brachytherapy requires a general anesthetic, the process of implanting the radioactive seeds is fairly minor.

Rates of incontinence can be lower for patients who undergo radiation compared to surgery, but radiation can still have unpleasant side effects such as other urinary symptoms and irritation of the rectum. In addition, external beam radiotherapy requires a significant time commitment, which may be difficult to schedule. However, the most important downside is that the prostate gland is not removed so it cannot be examined to see how serious your cancer is.

Radiation or Surgery? [**MORE DETAIL**]

Radiation and surgery appear to be equally effective in treating prostate cancer in certain patients and have similar 10-year survival rates. However, bear in mind that we don't know about survival beyond 10 years. Studies comparing surgery and radiation beyond 10 years appear to show that surgery works better but these studies involved older, less effective radiation techniques. We don't yet know about the long-term effectiveness of newer radiation treatments. Also, we still don't know if radiation works as well as surgery for more aggressive tumors.

External Beam Radiotherapy

This treatment approach involves directing radiation beams to the prostate using a device called a **linear accelerator**. Standard therapy consists of 10 to 15 minutes each day, 5 days a week, over a period of 7 to 8 weeks. Radiation is given in daily, low-dose bursts to give the healthy tissue surrounding the prostate a chance to recuperate. Cancerous tissue doesn't repair itself as quickly as normal tissue, so over time, the cancer cells cannot cope with the repeated bombardments and sustain so much damage that they are destroyed. The surrounding areas of normal tissue, however, do recover from the radiation damage.

Conformal Radiotherapy and IMRT

Conformal radiotherapy has added a new dimension to external beam radiotherapy. With the aid of computers, multiple radiation beams are made to "conform" to the shape of the prostate, which means that higher doses can be delivered safely to the cancer while sparing the surrounding tissues, especially the rectum and the bladder. The high-precision technology necessary for conformal radiotherapy (which is only available in some major radiation clinics) has led to an even further refinement: **intensity modulated radiotherapy (IMRT)**. With IMRT, the radiation oncologist can conform the radiation dose tightly around the prostate to an even greater degree than conformal radiotherapy, allowing for even greater sparing of normal tissues. IMRT also allows the oncologist to vary the amount of radiation administered to different places on the prostate. For example, an oncologist can focus a higher radiation dose on the prostate lobe with obvious tumors.

Brachytherapy

Opinions vary, but brachytherapy alone is often reserved for patients with low-risk tumors—i.e., those with a PSA below 10 ng/mL and a Gleason score of 6 or less (see pages 17–19 and 22–24). In men with more aggressive tumors, brachytherapy can be used in combination with hormones or beam therapy.

The procedure involves implanting about 100 radioactive "seeds," usually

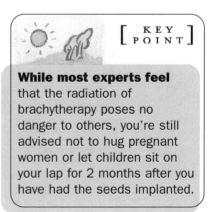

[KEY POINT]

While most experts feel that the radiation of brachytherapy poses no danger to others, you're still advised not to hug pregnant women or let children sit on your lap for 2 months after you have had the seeds implanted.

iodine or palladium, into the prostate through the skin between the anus and the base of the penis (the **perineum**). The seeds are positioned in the prostate using trans-rectal ultrasound guidance (see page 19), to lie approximately 5 mm (¼ inch) apart from each other. The radiation that comes from the seeds weakens significantly over a distance of only a few millimeters, so damage to nearby healthy tissues is limited, while the additive effect of numerous radioactive seeds results in a very high radiation dose being delivered to the prostate. Typically, the procedure can be done as a 1-day procedure and you do not have to stay in hospital overnight. Although the seeds are permanently implanted, their radioactivity only lasts a few months.

Prostate Cancer: The Case for Drug Therapy

About 50 years ago Charles Huggins, an American urologist, discovered that prostate cancer grows in response to male hormones (**androgens**), of which testosterone is the most important, and that reducing testosterone levels causes prostate cancer cells to regress. This discovery not only earned a Nobel Prize for Dr. Huggins, but also created an effective treatment for men whose prostate cancer had spread. There is now a wide range of treatments that shrink prostate cancer by interfering with testosterone.

Drug treatment is usually reserved for men who cannot have surgery or radiotherapy, for example, men whose prostate cancer has already metastasized beyond the prostate gland, or who have other medical conditions that rule out surgery or radiation. Drugs are also helpful after surgery or radiation as a preventive measure for very aggressive cancers, or as a treatment if the cancer returns.

The huge advantage of hormone medications for prostate cancer compared to "conventional" chemotherapy for other types of cancers is that these hormonal approaches target only testosterone—they do not affect other organs or body systems—so they are generally well-tolerated, regardless of whether you have other medical illnesses.

The downside of these drugs is that lack of testosterone can itself cause side effects, which you have to weigh against their life-saving effects. You may feel tired and fragile due to loss of muscle strength. **Osteoporosis** (brittle bones) and **anemia** (see page 58) are also long-term risks. Loss of libido and sexual function, hot flashes, and sweating are also common complaints.

LHRH Agonists

Luteinizing hormone-releasing hormone (LHRH) agonists are artificial versions of a natural hormone, luteinizing hormone-releasing hormone. They work by stimulating the **pituitary gland**, a small gland tucked underneath the brain, to produce a hormone called **luteinizing hormone (LH)**. At first this stimulates the testicles to produce more testosterone, but then a complex feedback mechanism kicks in that dampens down LH production and testosterone levels start to fall. Within about 3 weeks, testosterone levels in the body become almost undetectable and stay that way as long as therapy is continued.

LHRH agonists need to be given by injection under your skin or into a muscle by a nurse or physician every 1 to 4 months. LHRH agonists include goserelin (Zoladex), leuprolide (e.g., Lupron), and triptorelin (Trelstar Depot).

Antiandrogens

Another approach is to leave testosterone blood levels unchanged, but prevent testosterone from "switching on" the prostate cancer cells. **Antiandrogen** medications do this by blocking testosterone at the level of the prostate cancer cells. Like a false key in the ignition, they block the testosterone receptors on the outside of prostate cancer cells, preventing the testosterone "key" from entering.

Again, the advantage of this approach is that antiandrogens only target cells with testosterone receptors, so other body systems are not affected. Another benefit of antiandrogens is that they block the small amount of testosterone produced by the adrenal glands, which is not affected by LHRH agonists. Antiandrogens include bicalutamide (Casodex), flutamide (Eulexin), and nilutamide (Nilandron). They are sometimes used in combination with LHRH agonists.

Prostate Cancer: The Case for Surgery

Making the decision to have surgery can be hard, even if it seems like the best and most obvious course of action.

Surgery for prostate cancer is called **radical prostatectomy**. It involves complete removal of the prostate gland and the surrounding tissue, including a structure called the seminal vesicles that are attached to the prostate. For a detailed description of radical prostatectomy, see Chapter 6.

The operation takes 2 to 3 hours and you would stay in the hospital for about 2 days. You would be discharged with a catheter in place to drain your bladder, which would be removed by your surgeon 1 to 3 weeks after the procedure. It usually takes about 3 to 5 weeks to recover fully.

Help Yourself...
To the Right Surgeon

Your health care should be a partnership, so you must feel completely comfortable about your choice of surgeon. Radical prostatectomy is a major operation and considered technically difficult. A recent report published in the prestigious *New England Journal of Medicine* showed that patients suffered fewer complications when their surgeon had performed the procedure often (at least 33 times per year). Keep in mind that urologists are qualified to perform a wide variety of different surgical procedures and that radical prostatectomy is only one of many. Don't be shy. It's up to you to ask whether this is a procedure that your urologist performs frequently.

Advantages of a Radical Prostatectomy

One major advantage of radical prostatectomy is that we know it gives long-lasting control of prostate cancer. Current techniques have been around for more than 50 years and the procedure itself has been done for over 100 years—much longer than any other prostate cancer treatment. Repeated studies have shown that a high percentage of cancer patients have good long-term survival (20 years or more) after the procedure.

The other major advantage is that when the whole prostate gland is removed, a pathologist can examine the tumor in detail to see whether the cancer was confined to the prostate gland and whether all of the cancer was removed. With this information, your oncologist can determine if further treatment is needed. Knowing that the cancer was completely confined within the prostate can provide peace of mind.

Radical prostatectomy is now a more attractive option than it once was because of the arrival of improved techniques for sparing the nerves that control erections. You should discuss **nerve-sparing techniques** with your surgeon, although he or she will make the final decision on what is practical during the actual surgery, based on how extensive your cancer is.

When both nerves that control erections are spared, the probability of having erections after surgery is high—between 60 and 80 percent. However, bear in mind that this is an average. If you have other medical conditions that affect erections, such as diabetes, depression, or cardiovascular disease, the odds will be lower than this.

Disadvantages of a Radical Prostatectomy

The downside of radical prostatectomy is that it is a major operation and, like all surgeries, has risks associated with it. Remember that the risks given below are averages, and, depending on your own health, your own personal risks may be much lower (or higher). Your physician should discuss these risks with you.

Blood loss is the first downside to consider (see also pages 57-59). If your surgeon is experienced, your chance of requiring a blood transfusion, on average, is about 1 in 20. Blood loss, and the chance of having a blood transfusion, is greater if your surgeon is attempting a nerve-sparing procedure (see More Detail box above). The reason for this is that any attempts at controlling bleeding with heat or sutures could damage your nerves, so your surgeon, in effect, "spends" blood in order to make sure that your nerves are not damaged.

The risk of death during radical prostatectomy is low, about 4 to 9 in 1,000 patients. About 1 in 100 patients suffers a heart attack, bloods clots in the veins (which in rare cases move to the lungs), or similar "cardiovascular" problems.

Because the prostate is quite close to the rectum and is held in place by connective tissue, there's also a remote chance that the rectum could be injured. This complication is repaired on the spot and usually does not affect recovery time or bowel function.

Another problem that might develop after surgery is excessive scar-tissue formation where the bladder is re-connected to the urethra. This condition is called a **bladder neck stricture** and occurs in 2 to 10 percent of patients. A procedure done in your doctor's office, involving a small incision into the stricture, easily corrects this complication.

Erectile dysfunction is one of the most feared side effects of prostatectomy. Many men will experience at least temporary problems with erections after their surgery, although for most this is not permanent. If your erection nerves have been spared, you are less likely to have problems (see More Detail box on page 44). You are also more likely to have good erections after surgery if you had good erections before the operation. Some medications, such as those for high blood pressure or heart disease, can also affect your ability to achieve an erection and age can make a difference: the younger you are, the higher the probability that you will retain your erectile function. On the other hand, if one or more erection nerves had to be removed because the cancer had spread beyond the prostate, the likelihood of achieving erections after surgery will be lower. You are also less likely to have good erectile function after surgery if you have certain medical conditions such as diabetes, depression, or coronary artery disease.

Incontinence is another potential disadvantage of prostatectomy that you should consider (see also pages 96–100). Most men will experience at least temporary problems with incontinence after a

> "We clearly established the criteria: one, remove the cancer, two, retain urinary control, and three, retain sexual control."
>
> **Ron**

Prostate Cancer Treatment—Pros and Cons

Treatment	Advantages	Disadvantages
Watchful Waiting	• no invasive procedures • no drugs	• higher risk of metastases (cancer spreading) compared to surgery • not a cure
Radiation	• beam therapy is non-invasive • beam therapy doesn't require anesthesia	• mild fatigue is very common • beam therapy takes up to 8 weeks, 15 minutes a day, 5 days a week • anesthesia is necessary with brachytherapy • urinary symptoms due to irritation • bowel discomfort and bleeding • erectile dysfunction rates can be similar to surgery • can't check out the tumor because it's left in place
Hormone Treatments	• non-surgical option • may improve survival • effective alternative if surgery or radiation not possible • effective prevention for aggressive cancers	• not a cure • LHRH agonists need to be injected every 1 to 4 months • side effects of low testosterone include hot flashes, loss of libido, sexual dysfunction, fatigue, weakness • long-term risk of osteoporosis and anemia
Surgery (Radical Prostatectomy)	• still the "gold standard" for prostate cancer • one operation, lasting from 90 to 180 minutes • pathology report on whole prostate • greater certainty about cancer spread	• invasive procedure • potential for significant blood loss • general anesthesia is necessary • rarely, scar tissue build-up after surgery at join of bladder and urethra • catheter for up to 3 weeks • usually 6 weeks to recover fully • at least temporary urinary incontinence and erectile dysfunction

radical prostatectomy, but the odds of having permanent urinary control problems have fallen significantly in recent years—with new techniques to prevent damage to the urethra—and are now only about 1 in 100. The vast majority of men have complete urinary control once they recover from surgery, although a few will report mild leakage during coughing or laughing (called **stress incontinence**).

Finally, recovery from prostatectomy can be uncomfortable because you will have to live with a catheter coming out of your bladder through your penis for 1 to 2 weeks.

What Happens Next?

If you and your physician decide to go ahead with surgery, the next chapter will help get you ready to take this important step towards improving your health. If you decide that surgery isn't right for you, skip to Chapter 9 to find out how you can improve your long-term quality of life. You may also want to read Chapter 11 if you're curious to learn more about some of the medications you might be taking.

Chapter 4

getting ready for your surgery

What Happens in this Chapter

- Psyching up for surgery
- Pre-surgery arrangements
- The pre-admission clinic
- Giving consent
- Bowel preparation
- Blood transfusion options

You've weighed your options carefully and made a hard decision, but your work doesn't end there. Reading up on your procedure will help you to get organized and feel more prepared for your operation. Don't be afraid to ask lots of questions so that you're ready to face the challenge of what lies ahead. Once you've passed the physical exam at the pre-admission clinic, the next step is the surgery itself.

Getting Mentally Prepared

WELL, HERE YOU ARE—IN LINE FOR SURGERY. ALTHOUGH YOU'D probably rather get the operation over and done with quickly, you may have to wait a while before it's your turn. However, this period of waiting provides a great opportunity to get organized for the weeks ahead.

Get a Helping Hand

We know—you're tough and can handle a lot. But part of being strong is knowing when to accept help; this is one of those times. You'll need a trusted companion to accompany you to your appointments. This person can be your significant other, a close friend, or other family member. It's important to remember that you need to feel comfortable with the person who is coming with you, as many intimate details will be discussed at your appointments. The right person can offer moral support, help the time pass in the waiting room, and, most important, provide a second set of ears. Often, while you're engaged in the unfamiliar business of hospital protocols, you may miss important details or forget to ask a question you had in mind. Your companion can fill in the gaps and later confirm your own impressions of what was said at an appointment.

Once you've checked that your companion is available to come with you, it's important that you learn all you can about your procedure. Many people find that knowing more makes them less afraid of what's to come and helps them prepare for a more effective recovery. If you're reading this book, you've already started taking the next important step to psyching up for surgery. Whether you have BPH or prostate cancer, increase your knowledge about your particular condition and its treatment.

Learn from Others

Talking with other men who have undergone prostate surgery will confirm what you have learned from us and may help to reassure you further. If you have prostate cancer, you may also want to consider joining a prostate support group in your area: ask the local cancer society, or your community or university hospital.

"Don't be afraid to ask questions of your doctor. If your doctor is evasive or is not able or willing to answer your question then you simply run, don't walk, to the nearest exit and find yourself a physician that is. Don't be embarrassed to look for a second opinion. A urologist is a surgeon by background and will offer surgery where it might be applicable, but don't think that it's the only answer."

Ron

Ask Questions

It's also important to ask questions—lots of questions. There is no such thing as a dumb question when it comes to your health. Getting the answers you feel you need will give you more control over what's happening. While you're asking questions, feel free to verbalize your fears. It's normal to feel anxious about your surgery and talking about your worries can make you less fearful.

Take Notes

Another suggestion is to take notes. You'll be better prepared

Don't Be Afraid to Ask ✓

Here are some questions that you may want to ask before your surgery:

- O   How might this surgery help me?
- O   What might happen if I don't have it?
- O   What are the alternatives?
- O   How might the surgery affect my sex life?
- O   Will I have problems with urination after my surgery?
- O   What can I do to reduce my risk of having a blood transfusion?
- O   What other risks are there?
- O   Will I be given a general anesthetic or a regional anesthestic?
- O   (If you are having a radical prostatectomy) Is it possible to spare my nerves for erections?
- O   What should I bring with me to the hospital?
- O   How long will I be in the hospital?
- O   How long should I plan to take off work?
- O   Will I be in any pain after the surgery?

for appointments and tests if you keep track of important dates, contacts, and medical information. We've included a diary section at the end of this book to help you create your own personal medical history. Aside from jotting down your various appointments, tests, and treatments, be sure to include any other health conditions you may currently have and all the medications (herbal, prescription, and non-prescription) that you are taking. Making a note of your allergies and family history of serious illnesses is also helpful. Pull together your health-insurance papers and keep them with your journal; you'll need them to find out what expenses are covered by your insurance plan.

Pre-Surgery Arrangements

The time after your surgery is when you'll need help the most. Getting enough rest during your recovery is important for preventing complications and ensuring that you feel better faster. If you are responsible for household duties, it's a good idea to stock up on groceries and fill the freezer before your surgery. You should also arrange for friends or family to come and cut the grass or shovel snow for a few weeks after you come out of hospital.

After TURP, you should plan on taking off 1 week, or more if heavy lifting is involved. If you having a radical prostatectomy, you may need 3 to 6 weeks off work, depending on how strenuous your job is and how much heavy lifting is involved. If you have a sedentary office job, you may be able to return as early as 2 weeks, but even in this case, you should not engage in any activity more strenuous than walking for 6 weeks, after which you can resume full activity.

Pre-Admission Testing

Arguably, operating rooms are among the most exclusive and valuable pieces of real estate in the country, so it's not surprising that you have to fill out a lot of paperwork and undergo tests to qualify for entry. This all happens during pre-admission testing. It's an opportunity to get through the administration, have some tests, and learn about what's to come. You'll meet a nurse or physician's assistant, and possibly an anesthesiologist, and get answers to your questions. If there's one day you should really have this book and your companion with you, it's the day of your pre-admission tests.

The nurse or phyician's assistant will check if you use assistive devices, such as a walker, a brace, or a cane. If you live alone, he or she will discuss how you will manage everyday tasks at home after your surgery.

Next will come the usual array of tests that all people facing surgery must undergo: an electrocardiogram (ECG) to gauge heart function, a chest X-ray to check your lungs, and blood tests. The blood tests measure how well your blood carries oxygen (**hemoglobin**), your body maintains normal fluid balance (**electrolytes**), and your kidneys remove waste (**creatinine**). If you have heart problems, diabetes, or another ongoing health problem, you may be examined by another physician, such as a general internist. Be sure to tell your physician about *all* the medications you are taking, including over-the-counter drugs, such as vitamin E or anti-inflammatories (see Key Point box on page 54).

Meeting Your Anesthesiologist

Once you know you're having prostate surgery, you will meet with an anesthesiologist or nurse anesthetist to discuss the anesthetics he or she may use. If you've had surgery before, tell him or her about any past complications with anesthetics—or if anyone in your family has ever had problems with anesthetics—including a rare syndrome called **malignant hyperthermia**. This condition involves a rapid spike in temperature (sometimes exceeding 105°F) accompanied by severe muscle spasms.

Consent

You make decisions to take risks every day of your life. Some kind of risk is involved when you cross a road, place a bet on a horse, drive your car, or board an airplane. However, when you go into the hospital to have surgery, the risk you take feels different because you are allowing somebody else, usually a doctor, to make decisions for you. Nonetheless, it is a risk just like many other parts of life.

Although the doctor will be acting in your best interests, it is still important that you understand exactly what you are giving your permission for, or consent to. You are therefore entitled to know what is going to happen to you, why the procedure is needed, and what the risks are.

You may be asked for consent for your prostate surgery as soon as you agree to have the operation, in a pre-admission clinic or on the day of your procedure. If your hospital uses a formal consent form, it is important that you read it and understand what it is you are signing. If there is enough time, you can take the form home and bring it back on the day of your procedure. If you are worried about any part of the procedure, or you feel you have not received a clear answer on anything, now is the time to say so.

"It's tough to make your decision about how you're going to tackle it—what treatment you're going to go with and why. Once you've made all of those decisions, it's tough waiting for it to take place. I was very anxious; I was nine jumps ahead of the stick. I wasn't focusing on my work, hardly anything. Just wondering."

Jim

There are three types of consent:

Implied consent – usually reserved for minor procedures such as blood tests or having a tongue depressor put into your mouth. In these cases, you non-verbally comply by sticking your arm out or opening your mouth.

Verbal consent – can be used in an emergency situation, when there is no time to obtain a signature on a consent form.

Written consent – sometimes required before medical procedures that need an anesthetic because you will be given drugs that make you drowsy or put you to sleep. Some hospitals don't use a formal written form.

Eating and Drinking Before Surgery

If you're undergoing TURP, you will need to stop eating and drinking after midnight the night before your scheduled surgery.

If you're having radical prostatectomy, most surgeons require that you stop eating solid food 24 hours before your surgery and restrict yourself to clear fluids, such as ginger ale, tea without milk, clear broth, popsicles, and juice without pulp, until midnight before surgery. After midnight, you should not eat or drink anything at all.

Preparations for Radical Prostatectomy Only

Bowel Prep

There's a small chance that your rectum might be injured during prostate surgery, so to be on the safe side, most hospitals will require you to empty your bowels to reduce the risk of septic infection. This is done by taking a laxative or, more commonly, giving yourself an enema the night before the operation.

Aside from reducing the infection risk, there's another benefit to bowel prep. Because the anesthetics and narcotics administered during surgery tend to slow down your intestinal tract, empty bowels mean you won't feel too bloated or constipated in the days following your procedure. More importantly, you won't have to strain to have a bowel movement, which can be especially uncomfortable if you have an abdominal incision.

Blood Transfusions

The chances of requiring a blood transfusion during radical prostatectomy have fallen dramatically in recent years. If your physicians think you might need a blood transfusion, they will carefully consider its risks and benefits. The following are important principles of blood conservation, some of which need to be planned 4 to 6 weeks in advance of your surgery. You can also obtain reliable information on blood conservation from the American Association of Blood Banks (www.aabb.org) and from the American Red Cross (www.redcross.org).

Why Is a Transfusion Needed?

If you lose blood during your surgery, your hemoglobin level may fall and your body tissues may have trouble getting enough oxygen. This is called anemia and can lead to fatigue, a slow recovery, and impaired healing. A blood transfusion replenishes your hemoglobin and prevents this.

The amount of blood you lose will depend on a number of factors, including the size of your prostate gland (there is more bleeding with a large gland), whether your surgeon is using a "nerve-sparing" technique (see More Detail box on page 44), or other factors that may affect your health, such as your weight.

How Risky Is a Blood Transfusion?

In the U.S., a blood transfusion has never been safer. Blood is collected from healthy volunteers and tested for a wide range of viruses, including hepatitis B and C, and HIV. The risk of becoming infected with one of these viruses is now quite small (see Key Point box on page 60). Other common risks of blood transfusions are fever and itchiness, which occur in around 1 in 100 people and are easily treated. Rejection (hemolytic) reactions, caused by the incompatibility of the two blood types or your immune system responding to the donor blood, also occur, in around 1 in 500,000 people. These are mostly prevented by a special blood test before your surgery called cross-matching.

What Are Your Chances of a Transfusion?

Only about 5 to 10 percent of patients undergoing radical prostatectomy (1 in 10 to 1 in 20) need a blood transfusion after surgery. The single most important factor in needing a transfusion after surgery is anemia before surgery. This is one of the reasons your blood is tested before your prostate surgery, so that you and your physician can correct your anemia before you have your procedure.

Blood Conservation Strategies

Identifying and Treating Anemia

Treating anemia before surgery is one of the most important things you and your physician can do to reduce the chances of a blood transfusion. If your blood tests before surgery show that your hemoglobin is low, your physician may prescribe iron tablets, vitamins (e.g., B12 or folate), or injections of a hormone called **erythropoietin**. Erythropoietin is naturally secreted by the kidneys to stimulate the body to make more red blood cells and a synthetic version (epoetin alfa) will gradually correct your anemia by increasing the number of red blood cells in your body.

Donating Your Own Blood

Donating your own blood, or **autologous blood donation (ABD)**, is a very effective method for reducing your anxiety about receiving someone else's blood. It involves donating one unit of blood each time. Your blood is stored in the blood bank, reserved for your use, for up to 35 days. If your stored blood is not used by you, it is discarded.

You should talk to your physician at least 4 weeks before your surgery if you are interested in blood banking, but bear in mind it may not be available at your hospital or your surgeon may not recommend it for your operation if your risk of a blood transfusion is very low.

Donor blood transfusions
are potentially life-saving and
have never been safer. The risk
of HIV infection from donated
blood is now almost 1 in 2
million. The risk of hepatitis B
infection is around 1 in
140,000. By comparison, your
risk of dying in a motor-vehicle
accident is around 1 in 10,000.
Pre-donating blood may seem
like a safer option, but in fact it
increases your chances of having a blood transfusion—either
of your own blood or someone
else's—because you may
become anemic before
surgery.

Pre-donating blood may seem
an attractive option since it
reduces the risk that you will
need donor blood, but it does
have a number of disadvantages,
and you and your physician
should weigh these carefully
against the benefits. Despite the
careful storage and handling of
your pre-donated blood, there
is a (small) risk that it could
become infected with bacteria
that will be passed on to you.
There is also the small risk of
clerical error, so you could end
up receiving the wrong blood—
equivalent to having a regular
blood transfusion. The most
important downside to pre-
donating your own blood is that
it may cause anemia before sur-
gery and, if you do not receive your blood back, it may make you
anemic after surgery. Finally, it cannot guarantee that you will avoid
a regular blood transfusion—it simply reduces the risk by about 50
percent.

Planning Ahead

You should ask your surgeon, anesthesiologist, or both, about your blood conservation options as soon as you know that you are having surgery. If you are anemic, remember that taking your iron tablets as prescribed and eating an iron-rich diet may help reduce the risk of having a blood transfusion. Iron-rich foods include organ meats, turkey and chicken (dark meat), dried fruits, whole grain cereals, peas, beans, and dark green, leafy vegetables (e.g., spinach).

What Happens Next?

Once your questions have been answered, you've had the necessary tests, and have given your consent, you're ready for the next and most important step—the surgical procedure. Chapter 5 helps you prepare for the day of your operation.

> "I would tell people to get as much infomation as they can absorb, but no more–and be very careful about getting information from the Internet. There are some good sources, and some not-so-good sources."
>
> **Nat**

Chapter 5

the day of your surgery

What Happens in this Chapter

- What to pack
- Hospital admission
- Surgical prep
- In the operating room
- Tips for friends and family

Knowing what is going to happen on the day of your surgery can prevent a lot of anxiety and inconvenience later on. Once you're admitted to the hospital, you will be given a bed and a nurse will be assigned to look after you. Your medical team will do everything possible to help you relax and settle in. There may be a lot of waiting before your surgery, but when you're in the operating room, things will move along quickly.

What to Pack

THE HOSPITAL IS A BUSY PLACE AND THE STAFF THERE WON'T BE able to provide you with many of the necessities you'll need during your stay. It's important to bring:

- A bag with basic toiletries (hairbrush, shampoo, soap, razor, shaving cream, toothpaste, and toothbrush)   ◯

- A pair of roomy sweatpants with a flexible waistband for when you're discharged   ◯

- Assistive devices, such as a cane, braces, splints, prostheses   ◯

- Dentures, glasses, and hearing aids   ◯

- Magazines, crossword puzzles, or a good book to pass the time   ◯

- This book!   ◯

What you leave at home is as important as what you bring to the hospital. Unfortunately, there have been situations in every hospital where items have been misplaced, lost, or even stolen.

Don't bring:

- Money and credit cards

- Your watch or other jewelry

- A radio, a CD or tape player, or a cell phone

- Work (your time in the hospital should be reserved for resting and healing).

Gearing Up for Surgery

Most hospitals will admit you on the day of surgery about 2 hours before the scheduled operating time. Either your doctor's office or staff at the pre-admission clinic should have informed you about when and where to show up.

Once you've arrived at the hospital, a nurse or caregiver will get you prepared for surgery. If you haven't already signed a consent form (page 55), you'll need to do so before your operation. There may also be some other final paperwork. You'll be asked to remove dentures, hearing aids, glasses, or contact lenses. You may be asked to shower with a special antiseptic scrub before changing into a hospital gown. An identification band will be placed around your wrist; if you have allergies, you will get an additional color-coded band. If you're undergoing a prostatectomy,

"The surgeon was delayed because they were late getting the room serviced from an earlier surgery. So I was waiting around, lying on a stretcher for a couple hours waiting with my wife, chatting. Then they showed up and talked to us for about 15 minutes. They then wheeled me in and just asked me to hop from the stretcher onto the operating table."

Ron

Self-help on the Day

- To keep your mind off things, bring a book or magazine you've been meaning to read.
- Ask any questions you have *before* you go into the operating room.
- Give the following items to your companion for safekeeping: contact lenses, jewelry, eyeglasses, hearing aids, dentures, and other prostheses.

you may also be asked to wear **anti-embolic stockings** that decrease the risk of developing blood clots in your legs.

Either in the ward or in the surgical holding area, a nurse or an anesthesiologist will start an **intravenous (IV) drip** of fluids and antibiotics in your forearm. You may be given an injection of **heparin** to thin your blood and reduce the risk of blood clots.

In the Operating Room (OR)

From the ward, you'll be taken to the operating room holding area, a busy place full of hospital staff and other patients awaiting surgery. In some hospitals, people walk from the holding area into the operating room with an escort.

The operating room will likely feel cold. Your first impressions will be of very bright lights and a dizzying array of machines and instruments. The surgical staff will all be wearing scrubs, hats, and masks, and will be attending to different tasks. You'll lie down on a narrow operating table in the center of the room, where you will be strapped in to make sure you don't accidentally move out of place during the surgery. A blood-pressure cuff, as well as other monitoring devices, will be attached to your arm. An oxygen mask may be placed over your nose and mouth.

> "You get out of this waiting-room bed and you walk to your surgery. And I thought, that is the worst experience they could ever give a guy. And when I talk to guys they say, 'You know what, you're right, that happened to me—I thought I was abnormal,' and I say, 'You're not abnormal, every guy has to do it.'"
>
> **Jim**

Since TURP (trans-urethral resection of the prostate) is a shorter operation lasting about an hour, you could have a regional or general anesthetic.

Radical prostatectomy via the perineum or abdomen takes about 2 to 3 hours. If you are having a radical prostatectomy via **laparoscopy** (see More Detail box on page 75), this takes about 4 to 5 hours. If your surgeon takes a laparoscopic or perineal route, you will be put into a deep sleep with a general anesthetic and you won't remember the operation. Abdominal prostatectomy can be done using a regional or general anesthetic. For more on the choice of anesthetic, see the Key Point box on page 132.

Deep Vein Thrombosis

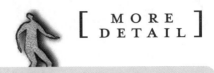

[**MORE DETAIL**]

The complete immobility brought on by anesthesia in both TURP and radical prostatectomy increases the risk of blood clots forming in the veins of the calf muscles. Under normal conditions, physical activity helps pump blood from the veins in the limbs back to the heart and lungs so that the red cells can be replenished with oxygen. Without the usual flushing action of movement, protein strands begin to collect along the inner walls of veins, trapping red blood cells and forming a clot or **thrombus**. This jam of protein fibres and blood cells can grow in size until it partially or completely clogs a vein (**thrombosis**).

Since three main veins drain the calf, thrombosis in one of them won't make too much of a difference. The usual symptom of this kind of partial blockage is calf pain when standing or walking that is typically relieved by rest and elevating the leg. Sometimes, excess fluid seeps from small blood vessels into the surrounding calf tissues, causing a swelling called **edema**. Because it is difficult to detect, staff in the recovery room and nursing ward routinely monitor for any sign of **deep vein thrombosis** (**DVT**). If the clot loosens and begins to circulate (called an **embolus**), it can become lodged in the main arteries of the lungs, which is a life-threatening medical emergency.

Although the risk is small (less than 1 in 100 in radical prostatectomy patients and even less in TURP), patients are given anti-clotting drugs prior to the operation and may be fitted with anti-embolic stockings that increase blood flow in the veins.

Friends and Family

Depending on your hospital's policy, friends and family members may be allowed to stay with you in the hospital ward. Their presence often helps to relieve anxiety, and they can provide you with support when you are giving your consent or asking questions. Friends and family will not be allowed to stay with you after your transfer to the operating room. There is usually a waiting area for them if they wish to stay in the hospital during your operation.

[**KEY POINT**]

If your friends and family do not want to stay in the waiting area, they should leave details of how they can they be reached in the unlikely event that a member of the surgical team wishes to speak with them during your surgery. Most surgeons also like to talk to family or friends after the operation to let them know how your operation went.

What Happens Next?

Next comes the main event—the actual surgery—although you won't remember much. In case you're curious about what happens during your operation, the next chapter gives you a detailed account of your procedure.

Chapter 6

the surgical procedures

What Happens in this Chapter
- The anesthesiologist's role
- Step-by-step guide to TURP
- Step-by-step guide to radical prostatectomy

The big moment has arrived. Your surgical team will do their best to fix the problem and start you on the road to feeling better. The anesthesiologist will continually monitor your vital signs once he or she has numbed you from the waist down or put you to sleep. The only things you'll be expected to do are breathe and lie still.

THE ANESTHESIOLOGIST MAY NOT BE THE SAME ONE YOU MET AT THE pre-admission tests, but he or she will consult your medical charts and history on the day of the surgery. The anesthesiologist will confirm whether you are having a regional anesthetic or a general anesthetic (see Key Point box on page 132).

Once you are on the operating room table, the anesthesiologist will use a number of devices to make sure your vital signs remain normal: a blood pressure cuff on your arm, four ECG electrodes to measure heart rhythm, and an **oximeter** that analyzes your blood oxygen levels by gently squeezing one of your fingers.

A General Anesthetic

For a general anesthetic, an oxygen mask is placed firmly over your nose. You'll be asked to breathe slowly and deeply for several minutes to ensure that you get maximum levels of oxygen in your bloodstream. The anesthesiologist will then inject drugs through your intravenous line that induce sleep. At first, you may experience some burning through your arm veins or a metallic taste in your mouth—these sensations are normal. Once you are completely asleep, a breathing tube is inserted into your windpipe.

A Regional Anesthetic

If you're having a regional anesthetic instead of a general anesthetic you will be numbed from the waist down but will not go to sleep. You will be asked to either turn to one side or sit up and bend forward as much as you can. This opens the space in your spine where a needle will be inserted. The skin on your lower mid-back is cleaned with an antiseptic solution and frozen with a small needle. After

Talk About It

Understandably, some people are quite nervous about receiving anesthetic, especially if it's their first time. It may help to talk to your anesthesiologist if you have any concerns before your operation. Rest assured that your anesthesiologist won't let the surgeon begin operating until you are numb or asleep, and will keep a close eye on you during the procedure.

that, another needle is inserted into your lower back so the anesthetic can be delivered to your spinal cord to numb you from the waist down. You'll then lie on your back again and your anesthesiologist will test the feeling in your legs to see if the anesthetic worked. You may also get some oxygen through a tube placed below your nose (**nasal prongs**).

Trans-Urethral Resection of the Prostate (TURP)

Once the anesthesiologist has numbed you from the waist down or put you to sleep, your feet will be positioned into stirrups—what surgeons call the **lithotomy position**—in order to access the prostate through your penis. Antiseptic cleaning solution is applied to your penis and the area around it. Sterile drapes are then placed over the area where the surgery will take place. If you are having a regional anesthetic, you'll be awake but you won't be aware of what's going on during the procedure because there will be a barrier draped across your midsection separating you from the surgical team.

Figure 6–1. Trans-Urethral Resection of the Prostate (TURP)

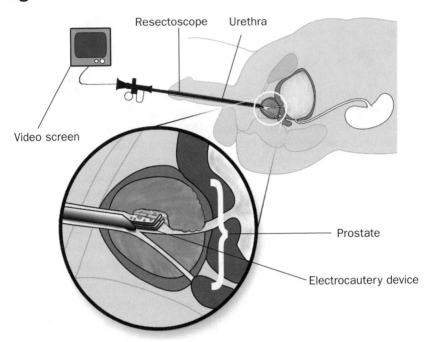

In TURP, an instrument called a resectoscope is inserted into the prostate through the urethra. The resectoscope contains a tiny camera that allows the surgeon to watch the procedure on a video screen. An electrocautery probe uses an electrical current to destroy the enlarged prostate tissue.

Your surgeon will begin by inserting a telescopic device called a **resectoscope** into your urethra (see Figure 6–1). A fiber-optic video camera connected to the resectoscope allows the surgical team to watch the procedure on a monitor screen. You may be able to watch the screen if you receive a regional anesthetic, but you don't have to watch if you don't want to. Once the resectoscope reaches your prostate, the obstructive tissue will be scraped out using **electrocautery**.

Electrocautery involves using a small probe charged with a

high-energy electrical current to burn away the obstructive prostate tissue. This device seals off local blood vessels as it goes through tissue to minimize bleeding. A **grounding pad** will have been taped to your thigh before your surgery starts to prevent electrical shock.

Once your surgeon is satisfied with the amount of prostate tissue removed, the resectoscope is taken out and a catheter is inserted into your bladder via your urethra. After TURP, your bladder may be continuously flushed with slightly salty water (called a **saline solution**) to prevent the blood from clotting in your bladder. This is done by attaching a bag of saline to one of your catheter ports. The catheter automatically drains your bladder through a second port into a urine bag. Once the procedure is over, you will be transferred to the **post-anesthetic care unit (PACU)** and your recovery can begin.

Figure 6–2. The Operating Room

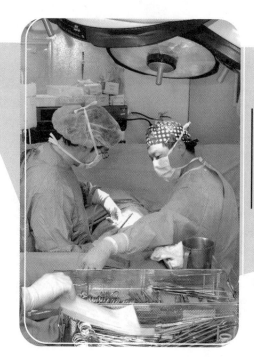

This is where you will have your prostate surgery.

Figure 6–3. Radical Prostatectomy

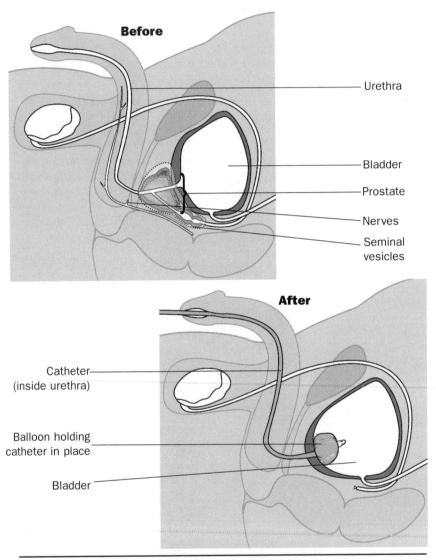

Before

Urethra

Bladder

Prostate

Nerves

Seminal vesicles

After

Catheter (inside urethra)

Balloon holding catheter in place

Bladder

Radical prostatectomy involves removing the entire prostate and the seminal vesicles. Afterward, the urethra is re-joined to the bladder and a catheter is inserted into the urethra to allow urine drainage.

There are a number of variations on how the prostate can be removed. Among them is the **perineal radical prostatectomy**, in which the incision site is the perineum, the area between the anus and the scrotum. Sometimes, resectoscopes and fiber-optic cameras are inserted through four small incisions in the lower abdomen. This **laparoscopic** approach takes twice as long as the standard procedure. Its minimally invasive nature could mean a faster recovery, although studies are still underway to find out whether it genuinely provides any benefits.

Radical Prostatectomy

Depending on your surgeon's preference, once you're asleep or your regional anethetic is working you will be placed on your back in one of three positions: the lithotomy position, as in TURP; an open-leg position, where your surgeon just spreads your legs apart; and the standard straight-leg position. All work equally well. Antiseptic cleaning solution will then be applied over your belly and down to your penis and scrotum. If you are awake you won't see anything, because a sterile drape is set up around the surgical field. As with TURP, an electrocautery grounding pad will be placed on your thigh.

An incision is usually made down your middle from below your belly button to your pubic bone although there are variations to this route of entry (see More Detail box above). No muscles are cut, which helps to minimize pain. A retractor is then placed in the incision to keep it open. There are six basic steps to a radical prostatectomy (see Figure 6–3):

1. The prostate is exposed and the connective tissue that holds it in place is cut away.

2. The **dorsal venous complex**, important blood vessels that sit directly on top of the prostate, must be tied off and cut to prevent bleeding.

3. Along the sides of the prostate run the nerves that control penile erection. During a nerve-sparing technique, these nerves are identified and separated from the prostate. However, if a non-nerve-sparing procedure is being done, the nerves are removed with the prostate.

4. An incision is made to divide the urethra where it joins the prostate.

5. The prostate and seminal vesicles are dissected off the bladder.

6. The bladder is re-attached with stitches to the urethra where the prostate once was.

When the bladder is reattached to the urethra, a catheter is put in place to bridge the new junction and will remain there for 1 to 3 weeks. Another plastic tube, called a **Jackson-Pratt drain**, is then anchored over the bladder-urethra junction. The drain tube lies outside of your body through a separate, small incision beside the main one and is secured with a stitch. The tube drains into an egg-shaped collector. This special collector continually sucks away any urine that might leak from the surgical join and cause infection. If urine doesn't leak (as is most often the case), the drain is usually removed within 1 to 2 days after the operation.

Depending on your surgeon's preference, the main incision is closed with either metal staples or sutures that dissolve on their own. A temporary dressing is applied over the incision and you're transferred to the post-anesthetic care unit (PACU).

What Happens Next?

If you've been under general anesthetic, you'll wake up in the PACU and then be returned to the ward. If you've had a regional anesthetic, you will be transferred to the ward from the PACU once your vital signs are stable. Now your healing can begin.

Chapter 7

when it's all over

What Happens in this Chapter

- What to expect when you wake up
- Your catheter
- A review of your other tubes
- Pain management
- Activities on the ward
- Going home

The first 24 to 48 hours after surgery are usually the toughest, but your medical team will make sure that your pain is under control and you're as comfortable as possible. You'll do lots of things to help your recovery along, such as breathing and coughing exercises, and taking short walks. Once you're able to eat and drink normally, and your surgical team feels that you are strong enough, you will be discharged.

The Immediate Aftermath

IMMEDIATELY AFTER YOUR SURGERY, YOU'LL BE transferred to the post-anethesia recovery unit or PACU. Although this clinical limbo can be a rather overwhelming place full of the strange sounds of monitoring equipment, hospital staff, and re-awakening surgery patients, most people don't remember much of their PACU experience. Waking up from anesthesia takes 1 to 3 hours, during which you'll experience moments of semi-consciousness followed by periods of deep sleep.

"I remember waking up in a daze. I felt okay, but I was in a daze. I don't recall any pain at any time, but there was some discomfort."

Jim

Return to the Ward

You'll feel groggy when you arrive back at your room. A nurse or caregiver will bathe you and take your vital signs (pulse, blood pressure, oxygen) to ensure that you're recovering as you should. You'll be given pain medication, made comfortable and instructed how to use the call bell should you need something.

If you feel nauseous or itchy, or experience a bladder spasm, let

Friends and Family

[**MORE DETAIL**]

Usually family members and visitors aren't allowed in the PACU. Typically, they may have to wait 2 to 4 hours before seeing you. However, your surgeon or a member of the surgery team will contact your family once the operation is over to let them know how everything went. Once your caregivers feel your vital signs are stable, you'll be transferred back to the nursing ward to complete your hospital recovery.

your nurse know so that he or she can make you feel better. Also, you'll likely feel thirsty and have a dry mouth, which can be relieved by applying some glycerine or ice chips to your lips and rinsing your mouth. However, if you've had a radical prostatectomy you won't be allowed to actually drink any water for about 12 hours, until your bowels have started to return to normal. After a TURP, you can drink water right away.

> "I remember my wife's words when I woke up: 'You're going to be fine. I talked to the doctor. You're going to be just dandy, he's got all the cancer out of you.' And that really set me feeling good."
>
> **Jim**

Your Catheter

After either TURP or a radical prostatectomy, you will have a **Foley catheter** coming out of your penis. This was inserted into your bladder through your urethra during the operation. The Foley catheter, named after its inventor, Dr. E.B. Foley, is a flexible tube, about 45 cm (18 inches) long, made of latex or silicone. It is often coated with hydrogel to make both its internal and external surfaces completely smooth.

If you underwent a TURP, the Foley catheter will be connected to three bags. Two bags hang on a pole, providing fluid that goes into your bladder to rinse out any bleeding that often occurs after TURP. The third bag drains the fluid and your urine, and hangs at the side of your bed.

The diameter of the catheter depends on the nature of the urine being drained. Usually a medium-sized catheter is chosen for prostate surgery, so there's enough room for tissue debris and blood clots to pass through it. A small balloon is attached to the end of the tube inserted into your bladder, which is then filled with sterile water. The balloon helps keep the catheter in place at the bladder neck. The exposed catheter tip is attached via tubes to the plastic urine bag by your bed. Special valves on the tube and bag allow them to be drained into a disposable container. Your surgeon may also use adhesive tape to place tension on the catheter, which will help stop the bleeding.

For TURP patients, the catheter is typically removed within 24 to 48 hours, before you leave the hospital. Radical prostatectomy patients need longer to heal, so they keep their catheter from 5 to 14 days, and leave hospital with the catheter in place.

Figure 7–1. A Foley Catheter

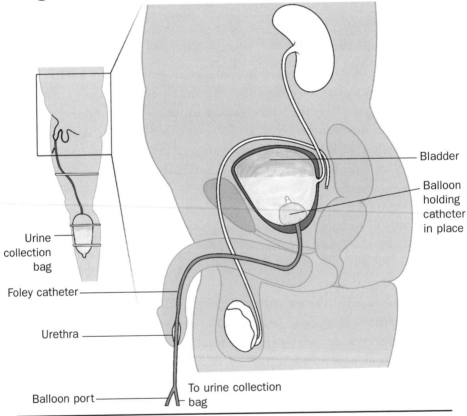

Bladder

Balloon holding catheter in place

Urine collection bag

Foley catheter

Urethra

Balloon port

To urine collection bag

For a while after your surgery, you will pass urine through a Foley catheter, a long, thin tube held in your bladder by means of a small balloon. The urine drains into a bag that hangs by your bed. Once you are mobile, the bag can be strapped to your leg underneath your pants.

Here's a quick summary of how all those tubes and other equipment are speeding your recovery.

What Is It?	What Does It Do?
Oxygen mask or nasal prongs	Helps you breathe
Intravenous line (from your arm)	Gives you pain medication, antibiotics, and fluids
Foley catheter (from your penis)	Allows urine, blood, and debris to drain from your bladder
TURP Only Continuous bladder irrigation equipment	Saline solution connected to the Foley catheter to rinse out your bladder
Radical Prostatectomy Only Jackson-Pratt drain tube	Drains fluid from site of surgery

The drainage from the catheter may appear quite bloody at first—don't be alarmed. This is normal. It only takes a few drops of blood to discolor a bag of urine.

Other Tubes

You'll slowly become aware of the other tubes and equipment that are still attached to you. You may have an oxygen mask or nasal prongs on your face to help you breathe. You will still have your intravenous line, which was inserted into your arm before your surgery. Through your

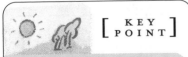

[KEY POINT]

If you've had a radical prostatectomy, you'll be responsible for caring for your catheter once you're at home. However, if your catheter is bothering you in the hospital, don't try to fix it yourself—always ask for assistance

line, your medical team will give you pain medication, possibly antibiotics, and fluids until you begin eating and drinking normally.

If you have had a radical prostatectomy, you may also have another line, **a central venous pressure (CVP) gauge**, in your neck, which your anesthesiologist used to monitor blood pressure during your surgery. If your CVP gauge is not removed at the end of your operation, it will be removed shortly afterward.

Another tube that you may notice after a prostatectomy (not a TURP) is the Jackson-Pratt drain in your abdomen. This drain tube is used to siphon away fluids that can accumulate around the surgical site.

Post-Operative Pain

"I realized it's far easier to keep pain under control than it is to react to pain—in other words to be proactive instead of reactive. For the first day or two I tended to ask for morphine almost by the clock as opposed to by the pain level, and it was administered. I slept well."

Ron

The key to getting through the pain after your surgery is, first, to understand what is causing it, and, second, to tell someone if you feel that your pain isn't under control. While some discomfort is to be expected after your operation, the pain should not be unbearable. If you are in too much pain, you may heal more slowly, so don't try to be brave or "tough it out."

If you had a general anesthetic, you may notice afterward that your throat is sore from the tube that was used to help you breathe during the operation.

After both TURP and radical prostatectomy, you'll become aware of discomfort from your incisions and your bladder. Bladder discomfort, which is caused by your bladder muscles going in to spasm, will feel like a strong urge to urinate, or a cramp-like sensation.

Pain Relief Medications

For pain relief you may be offered narcotics such as morphine and codeine, but increasingly a non-narcotic such as ketorolac (Toradol) is used instead. All these drugs can be given via your IV line, as tablets, or as a suppository. **Anticholinergic** tablets such as oxybutinin (Ditropan) can also be helpful for bladder spasms. Occasionally, radical prostatectomy patients are offered **patient-controlled analgesia (PCA)** (see below).

If you experience side effects from these drugs, don't hesitate to mention them to your nurse. For more on medication side effects, see Chapter 11.

Pain Control at the Touch of a Button

You may be offered a patient-controlled analgesia (PCA) pump. With PCA, a pump filled with pain medication is connected directly to your intravenous line or your regional anesthetic line in your back. The pain medication used when the pump is connected to your intravenous line is usually morphine. If the line in your back is connected to the pump, you will receive a local anesthetic. By pressing a button on this pump, you can give yourself an amount of medication specified by your doctor.

The PCA pump has a safety timer called a **lock-out**, so you won't overdose yourself. If you press the pump button during the lock-out time, you won't receive medicine because there is a limit to the amount of pain medication you can have. Once you press the button, the pain medicine should take 5 to 10 minutes to work.

Here is a list of do's and don'ts for your PCA pump:

DO

- press the button when you start to feel pain
- use the pump before you move or turn, do breathing and coughing exercises, or do anything that causes you pain

DO NOT

- wait until your pain is bad before using the pump
- let others press the button on your pump
- use the PCA for gas pain or bladder spasms
- press the button when you are comfortable and sleepy

Get Busy Healing

Although a stay in the hospital may sound boring, you'll actually be kept quite busy, working hard to help your recovery. One important task will be to breathe deeply and cough, up to 10 times every hour. These exercises expand your lungs and decrease the chance of fluid building up, and the risk of pneumonia. Breathing and coughing post-surgery are particularly important if you're a smoker or have other lung problems, such as asthma. It's normal for coughing to be uncomfortable, especially if you have abdominal incisions, so try holding a pillow to your abdomen to absorb some of the strain.

You'll also be asked to wiggle your toes, pump each foot up and down (as if you were using your car brakes), and bend and straighten your legs. These exercises improve your blood circulation and reduce the risk of blood clots.

The next step is to start walking. It's important to get up and moving because it improves your circulation and reduces the risk of deep vein thrombosis (see More Detail box on page 67). Depending on the time of your surgery and when you return to the nursing ward, you'll be taken for a short walk that evening or the next morning. The first time on your feet is the most difficult, but your nurse will help you get going. You'll probably feel dizzy and quickly fatigued. Slowly, as you get more and more rest, you'll begin to feel stronger and walking will become easy again.

A day or so after surgery you will have your first meal. This usually consists of dairy products such as yogurt, pudding, custard, creamy soup, and hot cereal. If you are lactose intolerant, you will be given clear fluids such as broth, Jell-O, juice, and ginger ale. If you can tolerate a fluid diet, you'll be allowed to start eating solid food.

> "I came out, and obviously I hurt a lot, but they gave me the proper drugs. They had me sitting in a chair the next morning, and I think I was even walking around a little bit by the next afternoon. Things progressed from there."
>
> **Nat**

Going Home

When you're discharged, your nurse will give you a set of instructions to follow for your recovery at home. If you have had a radical prostatectomy, you will be discharged with the catheter still in place, so it's a good idea to have your companion with you on the day of your discharge so that he or she can drive you home (and write down the nurse's instructions for you). After TURP, the catheter is usually removed before you leave the hospital, but it's still a good idea to have someone else do the driving.

Discharge Checklist

Use this discharge checklist to make sure you have everything you need for your recovery at home:

CHECKLIST—LEAVING THE HOSPITAL

- An appointment to have your staples or clips removed (if needed) ○
- Prescriptions for painkillers and any other medications (if needed) ○
- A contact name and number in case of an emergency ○
- A general information package, including a list of do's and don'ts ○
- Someone to escort you home ○
- A follow-up appointment ○
- Your personal items ○
- This book! ○

What Happens Next?

Once you're at home, it will be a time for you to rest and heal. If you had a radical prostatectomy, you'll need to learn to care for your surgical wound and catheter, and there will be at least one follow-up visit to the urologist. You'll also have to keep an eye out for complications or side effects from your surgery.

Chapter 8

recovering at home

What Happens in this Chapter

- Caring for a surgical incision
- Managing your catheter
- Exercise, driving, flying, work, sex
- Follow-up with your doctor
- Side effects of TURP and radical prostatectomy
- Treatments for incontinence
- Treatments for erectile dysfunction

The surgeon's job is over, but now it's your turn to take the lead. You'll be responsible for caring for your incisions and following up with your physician. Even though you'll have to exercise as part of your recovery, you'll still need plenty of rest and should return to your normal routine gradually. Most men experience urinary problems and sexual difficulties—at least temporarily—after a prostate procedure. There are several avenues open to you to deal with these common side effects of surgery.

Controlling Infection After Radical Prostatectomy

HUMAN BEINGS NORMALLY HARBOR VAST NUMBERS OF BACTERIA ON their skin, in their stomachs, and in moist openings such as the mouth, nose, anus, and urethra. Most are harmless and, in some cases, are essential for life itself. What's more, these less harmful bacteria take up space that might otherwise be colonized by more dangerous germs. Proper hygiene and a healthy immune system usually keep this microscopic "wild kingdom" in balance.

While infection of a surgical wound after prostate removal is rare, it does happen. It's slightly more of a challenge to keep your catheter infection-free for up to 2 weeks. Careful and diligent personal hygiene is a must to avoid the miseries of bladder and urinary tract infections. Therefore, before you leave the hospital, your nurse will give you a crash course on how to look after your incision and catheter.

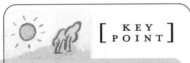

[**KEY POINT**]

Until your incisions have fully healed, keep the area clean with mild soapy water, rinse well, and pat dry. Avoid using talcum-type powders and skin lotions near your incisions because these products can trap bacteria.

Surgical Wound Care

If you're nervous about having to care for your incision, don't be. It's no different than caring for a regular cut. The key is to keep the wounded area as clean as possible. Since incision sites are often left open to the air during your recovery period, frequent hand-washing is the best way to avoid infection through contact. You can also feel free to shower regularly, even while your stitches are still in place. If your wound does become infected, you'll be prescribed antibiotics.

Your incision will be closed with either dissolvable stitches or surgical staples. Your stitches, which are under the skin and invisible, will be harmlessly absorbed by your body during the healing process and don't require a follow-up appointment. If the light, plastic tape that covers your stitches falls off in the shower the tape doesn't have to be replaced. If your surgeon used surgical staples you will have them removed either by your family doctor or a visiting nurse.

Catheter Care

While you were in the hospital, your nurse looked after your catheter. However, now it's your responsibility. Caring for your catheter is easy with a little practice and an understanding of how it works. A catheter uses gravity to drain urine from your bladder. So the first rule of living with a catheter is to always keep the drainage bag lower than your bladder. The bags come in two sizes. The smaller bag is for daytime activity and is attached securely to your upper thigh to reduce painful tugging on the catheter when you move. You can shower with the day-bag in place and it fits under track pants so that you can move around freely, which in turn promotes better drainage. The larger size is for overnight use and lies by the side of your bed.

In the same way that running water stays fresh, urine usually remains sterile if it is routinely drained from your bladder. However, if urine sits around for a long time, it quickly becomes a breeding ground for bacteria that can infect your bladder and urethra. Keep an eye out for kinks in the tubing, which can prevent your urine from flowing freely.

Another site that's vulnerable to infection is the **urethral meatus**, the opening where the catheter is inserted into your penis. Some urine normally bypasses around the catheter when you sneeze, cough, or have bowel movements, so strict hygiene is essential while you're living with your catheter. Gently cleanse the foreskin, the glans, the meatus, and the catheter with antiseptic cleaning solution or soapy water at least twice daily. Pat dry. Make sure whatever you use to clean these areas is disposable—don't use the same cloth, wipe, or towel more than once. Some doctors suggest applying a dab of antiseptic cream to the meatus as an additional precaution against infection.

Also, if you aren't circumcised, make sure the foreskin isn't retracted behind the glans for a long period of time because this can restrict blood flow and cause your glans to swell painfully. Clean new bags with warm water and a few drops of liquid soap or vinegar before using them, and let them drip dry. Always wash your hands before and after cleaning the area around your catheter or your catheter equipment.

You should try to drink 2 to 3 liters (32 to 48 oz) of fluid a day

[S E L F - H E L P]

Catheter Care as Easy as 1, 2, 3

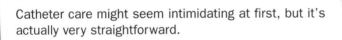

Catheter care might seem intimidating at first, but it's actually very straightforward.

1. Make sure your urine bag rests below your bladder.

2. Clean new urine bags before you use them, as well as the area around your catheter, including the foreskin, glans, and meatus. Be sure to wash your hands before and after.

3. Drink 2 to 3 liters (32 to 48 oz) of fluid each day to flush out your bladder.

to flush out your bladder. Water, tea, and juice are best. Typically, your urine should be clear yellow, but it can turn a pinkish color after too much activity, a bowel movement, or an occasional bladder spasm, all of which can cause minor bleeding. Call your doctor if your catheter accidentally comes out—a rare occurrence.

Return to Daily Activities

It's normal to tire easily after surgery, although the amount of fatigue varies from person to person. You're more likely to feel tired if you're older, so you may have to work a little harder to rebuild your stamina. It might help to eat frequent, small, high-fiber meals with plenty of fluids to make digestion easier and bowel movements less strenuous.

Exercise

For the first 3 weeks, exercise after TURP or a radical prostatectomy should be nothing more strenuous than walking. Start off with short walks and then progressively increase the distance as you gain your strength back. Rest when your body feels tired. Your recovery won't go faster if you push yourself too much. From about the fourth week after surgery, slowly return to your normal activities. Don't lift anything over 5 kg (10 lbs) for 4 to 6 weeks. You can go back to your sports activities after about 6 weeks, but increase your activity gradually and be guided by how well your body is tolerating the exercise.

Driving

After TURP or radical prostatectomy, you should avoid getting behind the wheel for 2 to 3 weeks, or longer if you still have a catheter, to allow the lingering after-effects of surgery and general anesthesia to resolve themselves.

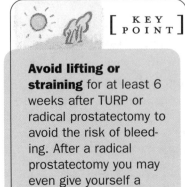
Return to Work

After TURP, you should be able to get back to work after 1 week, unless heavy lifting is required. In this case you may need a few weeks off.

After a radical prostatectomy, if you have a non-strenuous job with flexible hours, you should be able to get back to work after about 3 weeks. If your work involves strenuous activity such as heavy lifting or straining, you will need at least 6 weeks off.

Flying

Flying is possible within a few days after surgery, but bear in mind that after radical prostatectomy you will have a catheter, so you may wish to delay any trips until the catheter has been taken out. Remember, too, that you should avoid lifting and carrying heavy luggage for at least 6 weeks after your surgery.

Sex

After TURP, you can resume sexual activity 4 to 6 weeks after surgery. If you have an orgasm before this time you may experience some bleeding.

"It took me 6 weeks off work, but I was pretty much back to normal after a month."

Jim

After a radical prostatectomy, feel free to start sexual activity once your erections return. Some men can achieve an erection shortly after the catheter is removed but feel too tired to do anything about it. If your erection does not return, is not strong enough for penetration, or does not last long enough, there are several solutions that you can try. Unless your physician tells you otherwise, you will need to wait until at least 6 weeks after surgery before trying a medication for erectile dysfunction such as Viagra or Cialis. For more information on sexual dysfunction, see pages 100–103.

Follow-Up

Follow-up visits for TURP simply consist of a brief check-up with your urologist after 6 to 8 weeks.

After radical prostatectomy, a key part of your first follow-up appointment is removal of your catheter. Your urologist may choose when to see you based on how quickly he or she thinks your bladder will heal, or he or she may want to perform a **cystogram** before removing your catheter. For a cystogram, contrast dye is injected through your catheter into your bladder until it is full. A type of X-ray image is taken and then the dye is drained back through your catheter. If the dye leaks where the bladder and urethra have been reattached, then your catheter must remain until healing is complete.

You'll need to stop taking any medication for bladder spasms 1 day before having your catheter out because otherwise you might find it difficult to urinate (a condition called urinary retention). Catheter removal is usually simple. An empty syringe is attached to the catheter's balloon port (see Figure 7–1), and the balloon is deflated by sucking out the sterile water inside it. The catheter can then be gently removed.

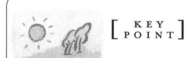

[**KEY POINT**]

You should be able to urinate within 4 hours after your catheter is removed, but let your doctor know if you can't. Frequent urination and a slight burning sensation are common—but temporary—symptoms after a catheter is removed.

Possible Side Effects of TURP

It's tough to contemplate the possibility of having side effects after surgery—especially if some of them could affect your sex life, or be permanent. On the other hand, many prostate surgery side effects are only temporary and occur rarely. We'll explore these together so that you'll be ready to recognize and deal with whatever you might experience.

Urinary Retention After TURP

About 10 to 15 percent of prostate patients are temporarily unable to urinate once the catheter is taken out after TURP, usually because the prostate gland has swollen or a blood clot is blocking the urethra. If this happens to you, you will need another catheter for a few days more until you have healed properly.

In rare cases, urinary retention may become a long-term problem, in which case the patient will be taught to help himself with a technique called intermittent self-catheterization (see page 33).

Incontinence After TURP

Permanent urinary incontinence is very rare after TURP (fewer than 1 in 100 cases) and most men regain full bladder control. If you do experience incontinent symptoms, these are most likely to take the form of stress or urge incontinence.

If this happens to you, your treatment options are Kegel exercises (see pages 97–98) or medication. Kegel exercises help your sphincter muscles regain their strength and are useful for stress incontinence. Urge incontinence can be treated with medications that relax the bladder to prevent spontaneous bladder contractions that could cause leakage.

Sexual Problems After TURP

Erectile Dysfunction

Erectile dysfunction is not common after TURP, affecting, at least temporarily, about 1 in 25 men after the procedure. If this happens to you, bear in mind that many things can affect your erections, including fatigue after surgery and anxiety. There is unlikely to be a physical reason for erectile dysfunction after TURP, and the chances are good that things will improve with time. However, if you find that your erectile dysfunction does not improve, there are solutions—see pages 102–103.

Retrograde Ejaculation

About 75 percent of men who undergo TURP experience retrograde ejaculation, in which ejaculate flows backward into the bladder, instead of down into the penis, during orgasm. This happens because the bladder no longer closes properly—either due to an injury to the bladder's sphincter muscle or damage to the nerves that control the sphincter. It is the most common side effect of TURP, but it is not a side effect of radical prostatectomy.

If this happens to you, you will notice that significantly less semen exits through your penis, and you may even experience a **dry climax** (orgasm without semen).

This condition is not dangerous, but it does affect your ability to father children. If you don't want to have any more children, retrograde ejaculation shouldn't concern you. If you still want to father children, mild problems can often be corrected with medications that improve muscle tone, such as ephedrine, pseudoephedrine, or imipramine. Unfortunately, if your retrograde ejaculation is the result of severe damage to the nerves or muscle of your bladder's neck, then the condition is likely permanent. In this case, fertility specialists can rescue semen from your urine for in vitro fertilization, in which your partner's egg is fertilized with your sperm in the laboratory, then re-implanted into her uterus.

Re-Growth of the Prostate

Occasionally a prostate will re-grow after TURP. This phenomenon is exceedingly rare and occurs many years (10 or more) after the original TURP procedure. This problem can be corrected with repeat surgery.

Possible Side Effects of Radical Prostatectomy

Urinary Difficulties After Radical Prostatectomy

Excess scar tissue may build up in the urethra or bladder neck and cause trouble with urination in about 2 to 10 percent of prostatectomy patients. This problem is fixed by inserting a fiber-optic device called a cystoscope through the urethra, allowing the doctor to see inside via an eyepiece. A variety of special instruments for grasping, cutting, and pushing aside scar tissue are then passed through extra channels in the cystoscope. Your physician may try to crush the scarred area to dilate, or widen, the urethra and promote better urine flow. Another option is to cut away scar tissue during a procedure called a **visual internal urethotomy**. Patients can be catheterized for a few days to a few weeks afterward.

Incontinence After Radical Prostatectomy

Virtually everyone leaks at first after a radical prostatectomy, to varying degrees. The good news is that the majority of men (90 percent) regain full bladder control in 6 to 12 weeks. About 10 percent of men have long-term incontinence, involving mild dribbling that may require absorbant pads off and on. Less than 1 percent of men have such severe incontinence that a surgical solution such as an artificial sphincter is needed.

A common reason for incontinence is that part of the internal sphincter muscle or bladder neck was removed. During healing, the bladder may become irritated or experience a spasm, causing uncontrollable urges to urinate (urge incontinence). Abrupt pressure of mechanical stresses on the bladder, such as sneezing, coughing, or laughing can also cause stress incontinence. Leakage can also be caused by an aging bladder that loses its muscle tone.

Non-Medical Treatment

For longer term, mild leakage, a non-medicinal treatment option is **Kegel exercises**, which strengthen the pelvic floor muscles surrounding the urethra (see Self Help box on page 98). Some studies show that Kegel exercises can cure the most common forms of incontinence after radical prostatectomy. You should notice an improvement in bladder control after 4 to 6 weeks. It's a good idea to start Kegel exercises before your surgery, so that they are already part of your routine when you return home. You can resume Kegel exercises once the catheter is removed after surgery.

If you are having trouble getting your incontinence under control, there is a wide array of disposable, absorbent pads and underwear that you can choose from. Finding a product that's effective and comfortable may take some trial and error. Believe it or not, you might want to consider disposable diapers for newborns. They are small enough to use as pads, very absorbent, and cost much less than adult incontinence products. Bring

"When I came out of the hospital, what really aggravated me was the leakage, the incontinence. But I became conscious of going to the washroom regularly, and every time I passed one I went—even if it was twice in an hour—and I retrained myself to stay dry."

Jim

Getting a Grip on Incontinence

Kegel exercises are a very effective treatment for incontinence after surgery. You can do them anywhere and any time while standing, sitting, or lying down. Wait until your catheter is removed before starting, otherwise they may bring on a painful bladder spasm or cause minor bleeding.

1. Find your pelvic muscle by trying to stop your flow of urine; the muscle you feel contract is the one you need to exercise.

2. Tighten this muscle as tightly as you can.

3. Tilt your pelvis forward. Tighten and hold the contraction for 10 seconds, then relax. The goal when flexing this internal muscle is to do so without tightening your abdominal muscles, buttocks, or inner thighs. It takes some practice, so be patient—you'll get the hang of it eventually.

4. Repeat 30 to 80 times daily, either all at once or spread out through the day.

an incontinence pad with you when you come to have your catheter removed, so you stay dry as you leave the appointment.

Medication

If your incontinence is persistent, there are some drugs your physician can prescribe to try and help you, although you should bear in mind that medications are rarely helpful with incontinence after radical prostatectomy. If your main problem is urge incontinence, several drugs can relieve cramps and spasms by

Buyer Beware!

[**MORE DETAIL**]

There are some incontinence products that should be avoided altogether, such as condom catheters and urethral clamps. The catheter consists of a latex sheath that is placed over the penis. The urine collected by the sheath then empties through a tube into a drainage bag. Urethral clamps work by tightening a ring over the penis to close the urethra. If a condom catheter or clamp is too tight, blood flow can be constricted, which causes painful swelling that's difficult to reverse. The clamps may also damage the urethra.

relaxing the bladder's detrusor muscle. These include the natural **belladonna alkaloids** (atropine, belladonna, hyoscyamine, and scopolamine), oxybutynin chloride (Ditropan), and tolterodine tartrate (Detrol). For more on incontinence, see Chapter 11.

Surgery

If your incontinence is particularly stubborn, there are a variety of surgical interventions that can help. The **male sling procedure** is emerging as an effective therapy for men with minor stress incontinence. This operation involves stretching a "sling" of tissue across the perineum to compress the urethra.

As a last resort, surgeons can implant an **artificial urinary sphincter**. This is necessary in less than 1 percent of patients with incontinence after surgery, but, when needed, it has a high success rate. The device consists of a silicone ring with an inflatable, fluid-filled cuff that is implanted around the urethra. This device can be extremely helpful, but mechanical problems and infection are possibilities.

Erectile Dysfunction After Radical Prostatectomy

Most men who undergo radical prostatectomy experience some erectile dysfunction, at least temporarily. They may be able to get an erection, but not strong enough for penetration; others may only be able to keep an erection for a short time.

Even if you are having difficulty achieving an erection, the sensitivity of your penis won't be affected, nor will your ability to achieve an orgasm. Most men can achieve orgasm without an erection by masturbation, although in this case there will be no ejaculate.

However, it is important to realize that for most men, erectile difficulties are not permanent. Avoiding permanent erectile dysfunction after surgery hinges on whether your surgeon can spare the two nerve pathways that control the blood vessels in the penis. These nerves are situated in a narrow channel between the prostate and the rectum. They act as "gatekeepers" that open the arteries in the penis so blood can fill its chambers. At the same time that these nerves are triggered, the veins in the penis are signaled to

"I can't get erections, I can't penetrate. But I've been married for over 30 years. I've got a great marriage. And I always say creativity...If a man's got a tongue and ten fingers he can be very creative and have sex...I still have orgasms, but I have dry orgasms. So my sex life right now is satisfactory."

Jim

constrict, which slows the flow of blood being drained away. The net result is that more blood flows in than out, so the penis gets stiff and stands erect. After orgasm, the nerves send a reverse message that makes the arteries constrict and the veins open up, and blood flows out of the penis.

There are now well-established surgical techniques for sparing the nerves that control erections. However, even if the cancer is contained within the prostate, your nerves may have to be removed if there is disease in an area close to these pathways. Unfortunately, your ability to have an erection will be permanently affected if both nerves are taken out.

If one or both nerves are spared, your erectile function may still take a year or more to come back. The reason for this is that the nerves can be bruised and nerves heal very slowly. Bruising of the nerves is the main reason for erectile dysfunction if both nerves have been spared.

Fortunately, there are a number of different treatment options, ranging from pills to pumps, for helping you get an erection by dilating the blood vessels in the penis and keeping the blood there. Feel free to try several and find out which one works best for you and your sexual partner.

[KEY POINT]

Bear in mind that many factors can contribute to erectile dysfunction, including natural aging, other illnesses (such as diabetes), fatigue, depression, prescription medications, alcohol—and anxiety about your erections! It does not automatically mean that there is surgical damage. If you continue to have difficulties after surgery, see your urologist about possible causes—and solutions.

Non-Drug Treatment for Erectile Dysfunction

The **vacuum erection device (VED)** is an effective solution for many men. This device consists of a plastic tube that seals around the penis, which is then connected to a pump. As the pump creates a vacuum around the penis, blood is drawn into the penis. A rubber ring around the base of the penis traps the blood. After sex, the ring is removed and the blood flows out.

Medications for Erectile Dysfunction

The treatment of erectile dysfunction was revolutionized in 1998 by the launch of sildenafil (known to millions as Viagra)—the first oral treatment for erectile dysfunction and one of the most intensively studied medications in history. Viagra was the first of a group of drugs called the **phosphodiesterase-5 (PDE5) inhibitors**, which work by encouraging blood flow in the spongy tissue of the penis upon sexual stimulation. New PDE5 inhibitors include tadalafil (Cialis) and vardenafil (Levitra). Your physician will be able to tell you if these drugs are available.

PDE5 inhibitors were a breakthrough because they do not automatically create erections—a sexual stimulus is needed. This means that you can take a tablet in anticipation of sex, but if the moment is not right, no erection occurs, unlike with the prostaglandins (see below). Viagra needs to be taken within 4 hours of anticipated sexual activity. Cialis appears to provide a longer window of opportunity (a day or more) and thus, potentially, more sexual spontaneity. On the other hand, side effects may also last longer.

All the PDE5 inhibitors seem to work equally well. In studies, Viagra had a 70 percent success rate in men with erectile dysfunction after nerve-sparing radical prostatectomy (i.e., 2 out of 3 of the men successfully had an erection). Side effects of the PDE5 inhibitors are generally mild and include headaches and a bluish tinge to your vision. However, they are extremely dangerous if taken with some cardiovascular medications such as nitrates. Your doctor can tell you whether or not PDE5 inhibitors are safe for you to use.

A therapy for erectile dysfunction that is popular among some men is alprostadil, a type of **prostaglandin**—a powerful promoter of blood flow. This therapy induces an erection within 5 to 20 minutes that lasts for up to an hour. There are two routes for alprostadil: injections directly into the spongy part of the penis (Caverject) and a tiny tablet that is inserted into the urethra and then massaged into the penis (MUSE). Although it's fast and effective, alprostadil is not without its downsides. It causes penis pain in one-third of men and you risk **priapism** (a painful, prolonged, inappropriate erection) if you accidentally overdose. It can also cause a sudden drop in blood pressure and fainting.

Surgery for Erectile Dysfunction

If all non-surgical options have been tried, some men elect to have penile implant surgery to achieve an erection. Discuss this option carefully with your urologist if you are considering it.

Rectal and Uretal Injury

Surgery is never without risks. Very rarely, during prostatectomy, the wall of the rectum may be opened slightly. This is usually due to excessive scar tissue that occasionally forms between the prostate and rectal wall after the prostate biopsy. In most cases, this isn't a serious complication and a few extra stitches during your surgery fixes the problem. You'll probably just take a bit longer to heal after your operation.

"Yes there is a range of options for erectile dysfunction if you want to go pursue it. Some of the guys turn around and say that they'd just rather not bother about it."

Sol

Cutting the ureter, one of two tubes that drain urine from the kidneys into the bladder, is also very rare, but a possibility. To correct this problem, your surgeon will insert a flexible tube, called a **stent**, along the entire length of the ureter and then stitch the ends of the cut ureter back together. The stent allows the ureter's tissues to heal by shielding them from urine and providing an internal, stabilizing support system.

What Happens Next?

You've come a long way and your physical healing is nearly complete. However, you may still have to make lifestyle changes and face the challenge of dealing with lingering worries. Chapter 9 gives you tips on how to achieve the long-term changes you need to make and the tools to deal with some of the feelings you might be having.

Chapter 9

how you can help yourself

What Happens in this Chapter

- Understanding and dealing with emotions
- Managing stress
- Relaxation techniques
- Exercise
- BPH and diet
- Prostate cancer and diet
- Rediscovering sex

Every man responds in his own way to the news of prostate disease and the turmoil it brings to his life. Change is hard at the best of times, let alone when it comes in the form of a chronic or life-threatening condition. Take heart from the fact that others have been there before you and there are lots of strategies for getting through this new phase of your life, such as finding support, learning to relax, and improving your diet. There are also complementary therapies you might want to try. Every life change can be an occasion for personal growth and renewal, for sorting out priorities and reflecting on what you value most, and prostate disease is no exception. Although this chapter deals mainly with prostate cancer, many of these tips and techniques are also helpful for benign prostate disease.

Managing Your Emotions

MANY MEN PRESENT THEMSELVES AS STRONG AND STOIC INDIVIDUALS. They tend to play down personal difficulties and setbacks to minimize the anxiety of those who rely on them. However, when you are coping with serious illness such as prostate cancer, this show of strength may not be in your best interests. Understanding your own feelings and sharing your needs openly with others is not weakness—it is the best way to tap into the strength of others around you.

Why Do I Feel This Way?

Most people like to be in control of their lives. Prostate cancer, or any chronic illness, can make you to feel that you are no longer in control. You may have feelings of denial, anger, helplessness, powerlessness, and confusion now that your future is more uncertain. In addition, you must cope with the fact that your illness is also causing emotional pain to those around you.

> "The more that I talked about it to different people, the more I found that people were giving me support and that was giving me strength."
>
> **Jim**

Communicate

Good communication is an important first step in managing your emotions. Communication allows you to dissipate your feelings by sharing them, and ask for help when you need it—both physical and psychological. Good communication also allows those around you to support you in the most appropriate way.

Stay Positive

We know this is easier said than done, but try your hardest to keep an upbeat attitude. A positive outlook can have a major impact on your health. It will give you a feeling of control and decrease feelings of helplessness, reducing anxiety and stress. If you're having negative feelings, you might find it helpful to name them, either out loud or to yourself—"I am feeling anxious about my surgery"—before turning them to more positive channels—"but I can't do anything about my surgery now, so I may as well just enjoy dinner with my family tonight."

Live for the Present

We tend not to live in the present. Most of us live in the future, living our lives ahead of ourselves—hours, even days or weeks, ahead. We concentrate on what we have to accomplish, so thoughts of the future are generally associated with feelings of anxiety: "What happens if I don't get to work on time?" "What if something goes wrong with the surgery?" "What if I can't pay my bills?" The list is endless.

Many of us also live in the past. A preoccupation with nostalgia is associated with mourning or sadness because we are concentrating on what we have lost—our youth, our opportunities, our loved ones.

Living in the past or future uses up much of our precious time and emotional energy, and drains the pleasure from the present. It is important to take possession of today and enjoy what we have here and now.

> "Just worry about today and getting through today, and forget about yesterday—it's gone. And don't worry about tomorrow because it'll come whether you're here or not."
>
> **Sol**

Support Groups

Prostate cancer survivors can provide excellent emotional support for those who have been newly diagnosed with the disease. They can truly understand the turmoil that you are experiencing. It is

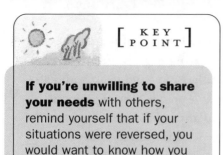
comforting to know that you are not alone, that many have traveled the same road before you and have had to make the same difficult decisions you are faced with. Many men say it is reassuring to hear a prostate cancer survivor say, "I've been there."

Professional Help

Don't forget that psychiatrists, psychologists, and professionally trained counselors can also provide emotional support and understanding in a confidential setting, especially if you find that you cannot talk to family or friends. Your physician or surgeon's office may be able to refer you to professionals who specialize in cancer patients.

"Sometimes my wife said to me, 'Well, you don't need to tell everybody about it,' and I said, 'Why not? I have nothing to be ashamed of.'"

Sol

Religion and Spirituality

Let's not forget what was the mainstay of stressed human beings long before psychiatrists and support groups—religion and spirituality. Many studies have shown that, in general, religious people manage life's stresses better than the non-religious and there have even been clinical trials demonstrating the power of prayer. Many men find that their faith, as well as prayer, aids in relaxation and decreases stress; others say they find comfort by speaking with their priest, rabbi, or other religious leader.

Managing Your Stress

Stress is a natural part of our lives—we cannot escape it. A serious illness such as prostate cancer is enormously stressful, but dealing with that stress may seem like the least of your worries right now. Nonetheless, it is worth taking a look at ways to reduce your stress because this will help with your recovery.

In biological terms, stress is designed to help us cope with short-term demands (such as escaping that saber-toothed tiger), not long-term demands. Long-term stress is exhausting, affects our emotional health, and wears down the immune system. This is not good for healthy people, and it is certainly not good for you. If you stay calm you will not only feel better physically, but will perceive things differently. You will be able to solve problems more effectively, view situations in context, and balance options. These skills are especially important when dealing with illness.

> "I was joking with people, saying they got me with my shorts down. Yeah, I was embarrassed, but I was happy to be alive. And I was happy because the people who were teasing me, and that I was teasing back, were people that were on my side, that had been very supportive."
>
> **Jim**

Invest in yourself by taking the time to learn some stress-reduction techniques. They will not take away the stress, but they will help you to manage it and prevent it from controlling your life.

In this section we briefly outline some stress-reduction techniques. There are also many self help books and tapes available on this subject. Just check out the "Self Help" section of your local bookstore or library, or Resources at the back of this book.

Relaxation Techniques

A good relaxation technique gives your body a chance to rest. By removing yourself from life's demands and letting go for a while, you will increase your feelings of well-being and control, decrease anxiety and panic, and help yourself face each day's challenges calmly. It may seem impossible to set aside some time for relaxation—with everything else you have to do!—but just one or two minutes a day is a good start.

Muscle Relaxation

When you are stressed you tense your muscles, so learning to relax your muscles, even under a lot of stress, is the most important first step. Relaxation tapes or CDs can help with this.

Start by sitting or lying somewhere comfortable and quiet, where you won't be disturbed. Close your eyes and focus on your breathing. Work toward slower, more regular breaths. Once you start to relax, concentrate on your head and imagine the tightness starting to ease. Continue to move down, repeating the process with your face muscles, neck, shoulders, and so on, all the way down to your toes. Feel yourself letting go, then continue to breathe regularly for a few more minutes.

Meditation

Meditation can be added to muscle relaxation. The goal is to quiet the mind but not empty it, so you may wish to think of meditation as a relaxation technique for your mind. At its most simple, meditation may involve repeating one positive word or phrase as you breathe in and out. As stressful thoughts intrude, they are acknowledged, then replaced by the word or phrase as you return to your mantra. Visualization (see page III) is a more elaborate form of meditation.

Visualization

There have been many studies showing the power of the mind in medicine. If you doubt that there is a mind-body link, try recalling a frightening experience that you had. You will find that your heart is racing once more and your palms are sweating. Imagine biting into a lemon—feel the saliva flow!

The goal of visualization is to harness the power of your imagination to help heal your body and encourage positive thoughts. This may be as simple as using images of lying on a beautiful warm beach to help you during relaxation, or imagining the colors of the rainbow, one by one, in time with your breathing. Or it could be more elaborate. One form of visualization, called **guided imagery**, can become quite involved; for example, you imagine your body undergoing surgery, then gradually healing. With **reminiscence therapy**, you focus on an event that gave you pleasure in the past and replay it in your mind.

Visualization is a powerful and increasingly popular technique, and there are many books, tapes and CDs available to help you explore it.

Sound Therapy

Listening to your favorite music can help clear your mind as well as being a good way to relax. Tapes or CDs of relaxing sounds such as falling rain, the ocean, or a bubbling brook also work well for many people.

Massage

Many people find a professional massage from a qualified massage therapist is a very good way to relieve stress by physically relaxing strained or aching muscles.

Loss of muscle mass and tone due to inactivity are serious concerns for older men who undergo prostate surgery. Just 12 to 24 hours in bed can make you weaker. So any form of movement—even shuffling around at home or taking short walks—is essential to maintain your strength during your recovery.

Exercise and Weight

Exercise is good for everyone. It will increase your energy level, help you sleep better, improve your cardiovascular system, and may even boost your psychological well-being by increasing your self-esteem and relieving stress.

Getting into shape is a good idea when preparing for surgery because it will help you recover faster. If you're not very athletic, get some guidance from your local YMCA, your family doctor, or a physiotherapist. It's never too late to start. Walking is an easy, inexpensive form of exercise.

If you are athletic, walking is still the only form of exercise that you should be doing for the first 3 weeks after surgery. You should be able to return to your normal exercise routine within 6 weeks after surgery, but build up gradually. It may take a few months to reach your pre-surgical stamina.

If you are overweight, you may consider shedding a few pounds before surgery. For example, losing just three kilos (10 lbs) takes tremendous pressure off your hips, knees, and feet, and reduces your risk of developing osteoarthritis. Getting rid of a large belly may also help relieve incontinence. We know this is easier said than done, but eating a well-balanced diet (see More Detail box on page 113) and getting more exercise may be all that's needed for you to reach a healthier weight.

Sleep

Lack of sleep adds to the stresses of the day and can lower your mood. You can improve your chances of a good night's rest by

- not having caffeine after 4 p.m.

- going to bed at the same time every night

- trying to sleep only when you're tired

- having a comfortable mattress

- buying some earplugs if your partner snores.

Benign Prostatic Hyperplasia and Diet

Although many food supplements and herbs claim to be good for prostate health, only one—**saw palmetto**—has so far passed the test of formal clinical studies. This herb has been described as the "old man's friend" and it has been used to treat BPH for centuries. Some studies have now shown saw palmetto to be effective in mild to moderate BPH. It seems to be as effective as (and work in a similar way to) the prescription drug finasteride (see pages 129–130). Vitamin E may also reduce the symptoms of BPH, although more studies need to be done to prove this.

What Is a Healthy Diet? **[MORE DETAIL]**

Diets are hard, so let's keep the rules simple. Try to eat less food that is high in fat, especially **saturated fat** (all those hamburgers and hot dogs), and increase your intake of fiber (fruit, vegetables, and whole grains).

Prostate Cancer and Diet

Several foods and food supplements may help you fight prostate cancer, although the scientific evidence is still preliminary at best. The University of Toronto Division of Urology recently conducted a review of scientific nutritional studies and came to the following conclusions about the links between diet and prostate cancer.

Vitamins

Although many people view vitamins as helpful, or at least, "benign," many vitamins can in fact cause serious harm at high doses. With vitamins, as with drugs, more is not always better. Always stick to recommended doses and avoid some vitamins altogether (see pages 115-116).

[**KEY POINT**]

It is essential to inform all people involved in your care about the supplements and over-the-counter medicines you are taking. A study that we conducted at the University of Toronto showed that 30 percent of patients with prostate cancer, or at high risk for prostate cancer, used some form of complementary therapy, but many of them did not want to inform their physician. Unfortunately, some were taking agents that were harmful to the prostate gland or made their prostate cancer worse. Tell your physician about supplements!

Vitamin E

There is some evidence that vitamin E may reduce your chances of dying from prostate cancer. The recommended dose is 400 to 800 IU per day and it is found in green leafy vegetables, asparagus, mangoes, wheat germ, whole grains, nuts and oils as well as supplements. Vitamin E should be stopped 7 to 10 days prior to surgery because it is also a blood thinner.

Plant Extracts

Lycopenes

Pigment-like substances found in plants called **lycopenes** are powerful antioxidants that prevent the cell damage that leads to cancer. They have been shown to inhibit the growth of prostate cancer cells in the laboratory. The hope is that lycopenes will prevent the spread of the cancer, but there is no evidence in humans as yet. Lycopenes are found in tomatoes, tomato juice, papaya, and watermelon.

Polyphenols

Another powerful group of antioxidants are natural chemicals called **polyphenols**, found in green tea. Like lycopenes, the polyphenols inhibit prostate cancer growth in the laboratory. Polyphenols can also be purchased as supplements.

Soy

Soy appears to inhibit the growth of prostate cancer cells in the laboratory, although again there is no evidence as yet that it does this in humans. The recommended dose is 40 grams a day. You can find soy protein in tofu, soy milk, soy powder, tempeh, or in the form of a supplement. If you are on a protein-restricted diet for medical reasons, it is important to consult your doctor prior to adding soy to your diet.

Alliums

These natural antioxidants found in garlic, leeks, chives, onions, and shallots also prevent the growth of prostate cancer cells in the laboratory and may stimulate the immune system.

What to Avoid

There are several supplements that you should avoid if you have prostate cancer because they may damage your health—or your wallet.

The Science of Complementary Therapies [M O R E   D E T A I L]

Complementary therapies are, generally speaking, not as widely researched as conventional drugs or surgeries and the studies that do exist are often not up to the standard of conventional drug trials. This means that we don't always know about side effects or how people with different diseases might be affected, so be cautious. A therapy isn't safe just because it's "natural" (the natural world contains some of our most powerful poisons). There are, however, a surprising number of good studies and the science of complementary therapies always makes for fascinating reading. For more on the link between diet and prostate disease, see Resources at the back of this book.

There is no scientific evidence that shark cartilage benefits anyone but its manufacturers. **Vitamin A** and **retinol** supplements can increase the risk of other types of cancers and should be avoided if you have prostate cancer. **Vitamin C** supplements do not appear to affect prostate cancer one way or the other.

Rediscovering Sex

One of the most difficult after-effects of surgery that you may have to face is impotence, or erectile dysfunction. Many men worry that their sex lives will be over if they are unable to have an erection. But remember, even if you're impotent, you'll still be able to experience sensation in your penis and have orgasms. Try not to think of erectile dysfunction as an end to your sexual pleasure—the way you go about making love will simply have to change. Communication is the key. Discuss the prospect of erectile dysfunction with your sexual

Get Creative!

Erectile dysfunction isn't an easy subject to discuss, but talking is the first step to relieving your fears before surgery or your frustration afterward. Here are some ideas on how to get a discussion going:

- Find a quiet, private place to talk.
- Make sure you have enough time to talk. You don't want to feel rushed.
- Start by expressing your own feelings. Don't make assumptions about how your partner might feel.
- Ask your partner to honestly share his or her viewpoint. Try not to be defensive if something your partner says upsets you.
- Come up with a plan of action in case you have erectile dysfunction. Figure out what treatments you might want to try and explore how you can alter your usual lovemaking to accommodate your condition. Be creative, get kinky, spice things up! There are lots of ways to be intimate besides sexual intercourse.

partner before your surgery (see Self Help box) and, if it becomes a reality, explore your options without embarrassment.

Remember, too, that your urologist can be a tremendous help. There are many medical methods, from simple drug therapies to advanced devices (see pages 102–103), to help you achieve an erection, and you should not hesitate to discuss the matter with him or her.

"I was impotent post-surgically. The surgeon deliberately went wide and took out both nerve bundles, so it was inevitable. You arrive at the position where you come finally to understand that love-making, or the passion of love, is brain-centered, not groin-centered."

Ron

What Happens Next?

Surviving an illness is a remarkable accomplishment. With a little effort on your part, you can maintain and even improve your good health. Check out the resources at the back of this book for more information on staying healthy. You may also want to read Chapter 11 to learn more about the medicines your doctor has prescribed.

Chapter 10

has my surgery worked?

What Happens in this Chapter

- Measuring success after surgery for BPH
- Measuring success after surgery for prostate cancer
- Do you need more cancer treatment?
- The role of PSA tests

After TURP, you and your surgeon will decide whether the operation was a success based on whether it improved your urinary symptoms. This may not be obvious until a few weeks after the procedure, when you have healed. After a radical prostatectomy, the pathologist's report may be able to tell you whether the surgery has removed all of your cancer. If cancer cells are still present, you may be offered further treatment such as radiation or hormones.

Has My TURP Worked?

Immediate Results

YOU WON'T KNOW WHETHER YOUR TURP HAS BEEN SUCCESSFUL until you are fully healed, so in the short term, your physician simply needs to find out before you go home if you can pass urine without difficulty and can completely empty your bladder.

In order to do this, your physician will give you a test called a **voiding trial** after the catheter is taken out, 1 to 3 days after your TURP. This is a fancy medical term for seeing whether you can urinate or not during the 6 hours or so after the catheter is removed. During this time, you may be encouraged to drink a lot of fluids.

Don't worry if you can't empty your bladder. Sometimes the inflammation and tissue swelling following the surgery can block the urinary passage until you are fully healed. If this happens, the catheter will be re-inserted to empty your bladder and your surgeon will either try another voiding trial in the hospital at a later time, or send you home with the catheter. The catheter will then be removed a few days or weeks after surgery, at which time another voiding trial will be done in the clinic.

If you are able to empty your bladder fully, you will be able to go home from the hospital without a catheter. To confirm that your bladder is empty, your nurse may use an ultrasound machine to check that there is no urine left behind once you have finished urinating.

After the catheter is removed, expect to see blood in your urine at first, but do not be alarmed—this will clear eventually. You may also experience burning or urinary frequency, but again, this will improve. Before you leave the hospital, you can be given a prescription for pain relief to deal with any discomfort, antibiotics to reduce the risk of getting an infection, and stool softners to stave off constipation.

Long-Term Results

You and your physician will decide whether your TURP has worked based on whether your urinary symptoms have improved. You may be asked to fill in another AUA symptom score (see More Detail box on page 15) to measure how much your symptoms have improved, if at all.

Your physician may also choose to perform some of the same tests that you had before the operation, such as a uroflow test (see page 14), for a "before and after" comparison. If you were having kidney problems due to obstructed urinary flow, he or she may also order blood tests to see if your kidney function has improved.

The surgery should have increased the strength of your urinary flow and reduced the amount of urinary frequency both during the day and during the night. Be prepared for the fact that frequency may not change right away. There may also be some urinary leakage for a few weeks while your tissues heal. If this continues for many months, consult your urologist.

Has My Radical Prostatectomy Worked?

When deciding whether your radical prostatectomy has worked, it is important to consider two issues: cancer control and quality of life.

Cancer Control

In order to decide whether your radical prostatectomy has successfully treated your cancer, the pathology report is key.

The Pathology Report

After your prostate is removed, it is sent to a laboratory where a pathologist examines your tumor and prostate tissue under the microscope and produces the pathology report. This examination can take a while (up to 4 weeks) because the prostate specimen needs to be properly prepared with chemicals and then sliced into very thin pieces before it can be examined.

As discussed in Chapter 2, by looking at your prostate in this way, the pathologist can determine the exact grade of the cancer and whether it is confined within the prostate gland. If the cancer is projecting outside the confines of the prostate gland it is more likely to have spread. If it is projecting to tissue just outside the prostate gland, the pathologist will determine whether the tumor has reached as far as the edge of the surgery (or **surgical margins**). If the margin is "positive," this may mean that tumor cells were left behind, although this is not always the case (see Figure 10–1).

The pathologist will also find out whether the cancer has invaded other structures by examining the seminal vesicles and the part of the prostate gland that joins with the bladder. If your pelvic lymph nodes were removed, he or she will also examine them for signs that the cancer has reached them.

"I found out by reading the pathology report that cancer was found at the surgical margins. About 20 months post-surgical, my PSA started to rise."

Ron

Once your oncologist has the pathology report, he or she will be able to tell you whether you need additional treatment for your prostate cancer and give you a reasonable prediction of your survival (**prognosis**).

Because you may have to wait a few weeks after your surgery for the pathology report, try not to think about it too much until then. Focus on recovering from the operation!

Figure 10–1. What Does Your Pathology Mean?

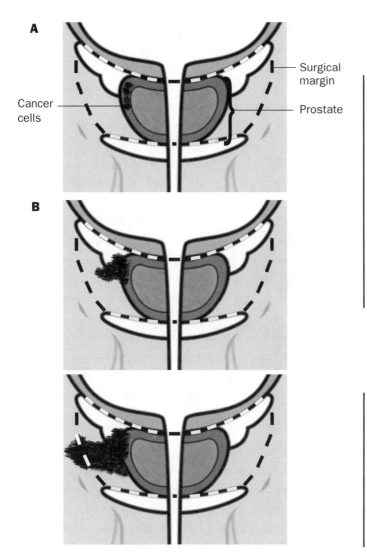

A

Cancer cells

Surgical margin

Prostate

Negative Margins
There are no cancer cells at the cut edges, so all the prostate cancer was removed. The tumor may be confined within the gland (A) or have spread outside the gland (B).

B

Positive Margins
There are cancer cells at the cut edges, so all the cancer may not have been removed.

Once the prostate and surrounding tissues have been taken out, a pathologist will examine them to see if all the cancer was removed.

Additional Treatment For Cancer

If your prostate cancer has spread outside the prostate gland, you may need some extra treatment such as radiation in the area where the prostate was removed or hormonal medication. This extra cancer treatment after surgery is called **adjuvant treatment** (see Chapter 3).

Opinions vary among experts as to the benefits of adjuvant treatment, so discuss your options carefully with your oncologist. Generally speaking, the decision usually hinges on whether your cancer has positive margins, how far your prostate cancer has spread, and to which organs.

If the margins are positive or if the cancer has definitely spread outside the prostate, your oncologist may recommend radiotherapy. If your cancer has invaded the seminal vesicles or pelvic lymph nodes, your oncologist may recommend hormonal treatments.

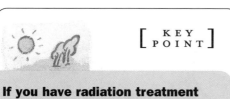

[KEY POINT]

If you have radiation treatment after surgery, the doses and duration of the radiation will be much lower than radiation that is given as primary therapy, and it is usually much more tolerable. It usually does not start until several months later, when you have recovered from your surgery.

The Role of PSA Tests

Even if the pathology report shows that your radical prostatectomy has removed all your cancer, your physician will want to keep an eye on you in case it returns. Regular PSA tests are the best way to do this. Because your prostate gland is the only organ that produces PSA, and your prostate has gone, all the PSA in your circulation should have gone too (see More Detail box on page 125).

What Does "Undetectable" PSA Mean?

[MORE DETAIL]

PSA levels in your blood will be undetectable after radical prostatectomy if all your cancer has gone. In practice, this may mean that your test results will say, for example, "less than 0.02 ng/mL" because this is the lowest limit that the particular lab can detect. Since it can take up to 6 weeks for all the PSA to disappear from your body after surgery, it is usually not checked before then. If you are unclear what your own PSA level means, don't leave your doctor's office until you are sure.

If your PSA never reaches undetectable limits after surgery or starts to go up, this means that there are still prostate cancer cells in your body producing PSA. The PSA could be coming from where your prostate used to be, or from other, tiny tumors that couldn't be detected before the operation (**micro-metastasis**). If this is the case, your oncologist will discuss with you whether to do nothing or whether you may need further treatments such as radiotherapy or hormonal therapy.

It is important to remember that PSA measurements should be done on a regular basis for the rest of your life. Your oncologist will be able to tell you how often they are needed.

Quality of Life

Quality of life is also an important consideration after radical prostatectomy, when you are deciding whether the surgery "worked" or not. Apart from the natural concern about whether your cancer has disappeared, the two most important factors after surgery that will affect your quality of life are urinary control and sexual function.

When the catheter is first removed you will almost certainly leak urine and will need pads to protect your clothes. However, over the next few months your urinary control will gradually improve, especially if you do pelvic floor exercises regularly to build up your sphincter muscles (see Self Help box on page 98). The majority of men have normal control of their urinary function by 3 to 6 months after surgery, although it may take as long as 2 years in a small minority.

If you continue to leak urine beyond this time and things show no sign of improving, you should discuss this with your oncologist, as there are several options that he or she can offer you (see pages 96–100).

With regard to sexual function, you will no longer be able to have erections if the nerves for erections were intentionally removed with the prostate gland during the surgery. However, if one or both nerves were spared, then your erections can start to return as early as a few weeks after surgery, especially once your catheter is taken out. Bear in mind that erections, like urinary control, can take a long time to recover—as long as two years in some men. (For more on erectile dysfunction and treatment options, see pages 100–103.)

What Happens Next?

Life after surgery can be a difficult adjustment at first, but be assured that, over time, most men find that their lives improve dramatically. Don't forget that your urologist, your oncologist, and other members of your health care team are there to help, so don't hesitate to call on them. Remember, too, that you yourself are part of the team, so take a look at Chapter 9 for ways you can help yourself make the most of your new life.

"Eight weeks after the surgery, my wife and I boarded the plane to Ecuador, and then flew out to the Galapagos. So there we were touring around, doing a lot of swimming and climbing around in rubber boats, and apart from the fact that my main piece of luggage was a lot of pads, I was feeling pretty well. I was back to work at 6 weeks, and off to the Galapagos in eight."

Nat

Chapter 11

medications

What Happens in this Chapter

- Medicines for benign prostate disease
- Hormone treatments for prostate cancer
- Medications before surgery
- General anesthetics and regional anesthetics
- Drugs after surgery
- Drugs for treating incontinence and erectile dysfunction
- Side effects

If you decide that surgery is not an option for your prostate disease, your physician can draw on a wide range of drugs to help you. If surgery is the next step, medications will play an important part both during your hospital visit and afterward, from the drugs that prepare you for your procedure to those that help you recover from the after-effects. You are the most important member of your own care team, and never more so than when it comes to medications. You should always be clear on why you are taking each medicine, how to take it correctly, and the possible side effects, so that you can help your physician find the best combination for you.

Medications for Benign Prostate Enlargement

THE PROSTATE IS MADE UP OF MUSCLE FIBERS AND GLANDULAR
cells. Both types of tissue enlarge and multiply as the prostate
grows, so medications for prostate symptoms fall into two groups:
drugs that relax the prostate's muscle tissue (**alpha blockers**), and
drugs that shrink the glandular tissue (**5-alpha-reductase
inhibitors**).

Alpha Blockers

As we discussed in Chapter I, as the prostate enlarges, the muscular
fibers in the gland become larger and squeeze the urethra more
tightly (see Figure I–4). Alpha blockers relax these muscle fibers,
allowing urine to flow along the urethra more easily. Studies show
that they improve both the symptoms of prostate disease and the
actual measurable urine flow. The downside of alpha blockers is that
they started out as blood-pressure-lowering drugs and can cause
symptoms such as faintness and dizziness. However, a newer genera-
tion of alpha blockers such as tamsulosin (Flomax), and alfuzosin
(Xatral) appear to target the prostate more than the blood vessels
and thus are just as effective but cause less dizziness. Alfuzosin
appears to have a better side-effect profile than tamsulosin. The
advantage of alpha blockers is that they work fast.

5-alpha-reductase Inhibitors

These medicines shrink the prostate by targeting its glandular tissue.
They do this by blocking the production of the hormone
dihydrotestosterone (**DHT**). This "high-octane" version of
testosterone appears to encourage glandular cells in the prostate to
grow and multiply. There are several 5-alpha-reductase inhibitors in
development, and finasteride (Proscar) and dutasteride (Avodart) are
currently available as medicines.

Finasteride appears to be most helpful for men who have very large, mainly glandular prostates. In these men, Proscar can reduce prostate volume by up to 20 percent and reduce the risk of needing surgery by half (from 8 to 4 percent). The downside of Proscar is that it can take up to 6 months to provide relief and does not appear to be as effective as the alpha blockers in improving symptoms and urinary flow. Dutasteride is a more potent inhibitor of DHT and works more quickly, reducing DHT by about 90 percent within a few weeks. Because DHT has few functions outside the prostate, Proscar and Avodart have few side effects. Sexual dysfunction (low sexual drive, impotence, and decreased ejaculation) is the main one, and affects about 3 percent of men, although this improves over the first year in about half of men treated. (See also pages 31–32 for a discussion of 5-alpha-reductase inhibitors and alpha blockers.)

Medications for Cancer

Prostate cancer is not treated with "conventional" chemotherapy cancer drugs. The idea behind drug treatments for prostate cancer is to "starve" prostate cancer cells of the hormone testosterone because these cells need testosterone to grow and develop. Although the medications do not eradicate the cancer entirely they can shrink the tumor and suppress the cancer very effectively.

The two groups of hormonal drugs that shrink prostate cancer are LHRH agonists and antiandrogens. Because these drugs are an important alternative to surgery, they are discussed in detail in Chapter 3 (see pages 41–42).

Anemia Therapy

If you are anemic before surgery, for several weeks beforehand you may be given iron tablets, vitamins (e.g., B12 or folate), or injections of synthetic erythropoietin (Procrit), a hormone that stimulates your body to make more red blood cells. After radical prostatectomy, you may be given iron tablets for a few months to help your hemoglobin levels recover faster.

Once you're in the hospital for your surgery, you'll be given two new types of medication that each serve a different purpose: sedatives and antibiotics.

Sedatives

Your anesthesiologist may give you a sedative right before you're taken to the operating room. The purpose of a sedative is to help you feel more relaxed.

Antibiotics

You will also receive antibiotics intravenously (through a vein) before your operation to prevent infection during and after surgery. These antibiotics will be continued for about 24 hours (depending on your hospital's protocol) after your operation. It's important to tell your doctor or nurse if you are allergic to any antibiotics.

A General Anesthetic

General anesthetics, which are given through a vein (intravenously) and as a gas, do more than just put you to sleep. They also help with pain control, relax your muscles, and cause amnesia (loss of memory), allowing you to forget events immediately before and after your surgery.

The dosing for your anesthetics will be carefully calculated and adjusted based on your age, weight, past medical history, and anticipated length of surgery. During surgery your anesthesiologist will make careful adjustments to your general anesthetics based on how you are responding. When you wake up, you may experience side effects such as nausea, vomiting, disorientation, and headache, although this is relatively uncommon. If they happen to you, such side effects can be effectively treated and should go away within the first 24 hours after surgery.

$\begin{bmatrix} \text{KEY} \\ \text{POINT} \end{bmatrix}$

You may be given a choice of a general anesthetic or a regional anesthetic. A general anesthetic puts you to sleep, while a regional anesthetic numbs you from the waist down as you stay awake. The choice of which anesthetic you have for your procedure will depend on your general health and any medications that you are taking, but personal preference is also a factor. However, it is ultimately the anesthesiologist's responsibility to judge which anesthetic is best; in general, the more medical problems you have, the more likely it is that you will be strongly advised to opt for "a regional" rather than "a general."

General anesthetics have evolved greatly since they were first used. There are now many different anesthetic drugs that provide a more controllable and safer kind of general anesthetic experience. The stages of anesthesia can be broken down into **induction**, **maintenance**, **reversal**, and **recovery**.

Induction is the period in which you are "put to sleep," most commonly with an intravenous drug. The maintenance period covers the time when the actual surgery takes place. Your anesthesiologist uses a combination of drugs to keep you asleep, relaxed, and pain-free, either through your mask or intravenously. During reversal, special drugs are used to reverse the effects of anesthesia and wake you up. During the recovery phase you are monitored closely to make sure that all is well as you wake up.

A Regional Anesthetic

Some TURP and radical prostatectomy patients have a regional anesthetic instead of a general anesthetic. A regional numbs the body from the waist down, while you stay awake, by bathing the nerves of the spine with anesthetic drugs. For more on having a regional anesthetic, see pages 70–71.

Medications After Your Surgery

Pain Relievers

After your surgery you will be offered pain relief such as ketorolac (Toradol), an anti-inflammatory drug, or a narcotic such as morphine (although narcotics are becoming increasingly uncommon). Pain control is an important part of your hospital stay, so it is covered in detail in Chapter 7.

Drugs for Bladder Spasm

Some men may experience bladder spasms while the catheter is in place after surgery due to the catheter irritating the muscles of the bladder. The spasm may feel like a strong urge to urinate, or you may experience actual pain. There are a number of drugs that can help with this, including **anticholinergic** drugs such as oxybutynin (Ditropan), taken by mouth, and opium and belladonna suppositories, administered into the rectum. A new drug called tolterodine (Detrol) is also for bladder spams. Medication for bladder spasms should be stopped 24 hours before the catheter is removed. Side effects of these drugs may include blurred vision, drowsiness, and dry mouth.

Anti-emetics

Some of the medications you receive for controlling your pain after surgery may cause nausea and vomiting. There are a number of drugs available to help with this, such as dimenhydrinate (Gravol), prochlorperazine (Stemetil), and granisetron (Kytril), which can be taken orally or given through your intravenous line. Side effects of these drugs may include dizziness, drowsiness, and dry mouth.

Stool Softeners/Laxatives

Stool softeners are prescribed after surgery to prevent constipation. A number of factors, such as a low-fiber diet, immobilization, pain control drugs, and the surgery itself can cause constipation. Laxatives, which work by relaxing the bowel, will usually be prescribed for you for 1 to 2 weeks once you are home.

Medications for Incontinence

Medications designed to help reduce bladder spasm—oxybutynin and tolterodine—can also reduce leakage and the frequent, urgent need to urinate, if this is caused by an overactive bladder. The side effects of these drugs—symptoms such as dry mouth, blurred vision, and palpitations—appear to be less common with tolterodine. They also cannot be used in people with any type of bladder obstruction, so they are not suitable for men with enlarged prostates, and are also ineffective for incontinence after radical prostatectomy in most men.

Medications for Erectile Dysfunction

Erectile dysfunction drugs fall into two main categories: those that rapidly create an erection (e.g., alprostadil) and those that allow an erection to happen if you are sexually stimulated (e.g., Viagra). Because these drugs are used to treat the side effects of surgery, they are covered in detail on pages 102 to 103.

Coping with Side Effects

All drugs have the potential to cause side effects. The goal is to avoid side effects or keep them to a minimum. Your physician can also prescribe or recommend extra medication to help you cope with some of them. For example, he or she may suggest stool softeners or laxatives (see above) to deal with the constipation that comes with pain-relieving medication. Increasing the dose of a drug gradually often reduces the risk of side effects. To find out more about the downsides of your drugs, read the information that comes with your medication or ask your pharmacist or physician.

Medications and Potential Side Effects

Drugs	Common side effects
Medications for Benign Prostate Disease	
Alpha Blockers e.g., doxazosin (Cardura), prazosin (minipress), tamsulosin (Flomax), terazosin (Hytrin)	dizziness or faintness after rising from a lying or sitting position, headaches, nausea, heart palpitations, stuffy nose, tiredness or weakness **RARELY** – heart failure and stroke
5-alpha-reductase Inhibitors e.g., dutasteride (Avodart), finasteride (Proscar)	erectile dysfunction, loss of libido, ejaculation disorder
Hormones for Prostate Cancer	
LHRH Agonists e.g., goserelin (Zoladex), leuprolide (Lupron, Viadur, Eligard), triptorelin (Trelstar Depot)	hot flashes, sweating, erectile dysfunction, shrinkage of testicles
Antiandrogens e.g., bicalutamide (Casodex), flutamide (Eulexin); nilutamide (Nilandron)	hot flashes, itching, dry skin, breast tenderness, diarrhea, nausea, vomiting, erectile dysfunction, loss of libido, breast growth, night vision problems
Medications for Surgery	
Anemia Therapy e.g., erythropoietin (Procrit), iron tablets: ferrous fumarate, ferrous gluconate, ferrous sulfate	**Erythropoietin:** heart problems, infections, nausea, high or low blood pressure **Iron tablets:** constipation, diarrhea
Antibiotics e.g., cefamandole (Mandol), cefazolin (Ancef), cefuroxime (Ceftin), vancomycin (Vancocin)	diarrhea, oral thrush, nausea, vomiting, stomach cramps, skin rash, kidney problems (gentamycin)
Anticoagulants e.g., heparin, warfarin (Coumadin)	stomach pain, hair loss, blurred vision, rash, hives, itching, loss of appetite, diarrhea, skin discoloration, bruising

Drugs	Common side effects
Anti-emetics e.g., dimenhydrinate (Gravol), granisetron (Kytril), prochlorperazine (Stemetil)	**Dimenhydrinate:** drowsiness, dizziness, dry mouth **Prochlorperazine:** nervous symptoms, twitching, tremor, shaking **Granisetron:** headache, weakness, fatigue, stomach problems
Drugs for Bladder Spasms e.g., opium and belladonna suppositories, oxybutynin (Ditropan), tolterodine (Detrol)	dry mouth, blurred vision, dry skin, constipation, drowsiness, heart beat irregularities, nausea
General Anesthetics e.g., midazolam (Versed), pancuronium (Pavulon)	nausea, vomiting, disorientation, headache for up to 24 hours
Pain Relievers e.g., Narcotics: acetaminophen+codeine (Tylenol #3), acetaminophen+oxycodone (Percocet), morphine; non-narcotics: ketorolac (Toradol)	**Narcotics:** dizziness, lightheadedness, nausea, vomiting, dry mouth, constipation, drowsiness, disorientation, skin rash, sweating, low blood pressure, shallow breathing **Ketorolac:** stomach and intestinal bleeding
Stool Softeners e.g., bisacodyl (Dulcolax), docusate calcium, docusate sodium (Senokot-S, Colace, Surfak)	**RARELY** – abdominal discomfort, nausea, diarrhea
Incontinence Therapy	
Smooth Muscle Relaxants e.g., oxybutynin (Ditropan), tolterodine (Detrol)	dry mouth, blurred vision, dry skin, constipation, drowsiness, heart beat irregularities, nausea
Erectile Dysfunction Therapy	
PDE5 Inhibitors e.g., sildenafil (Viagra), tadalafil (Cialis), vardenafil (Levitra)	headache, flushing, gastrointestinal upset, nasal congestion
Prostaglandins e.g., alprostadil (MUSE, Caverject)	bruising (Caverject), penile pain, prolonged erection (four hours or more)

What Happens Next?

It's surprising how many people don't fill their prescriptions for medications that can make a huge difference to their health. If you have concerns about something your doctor has prescribed, or if you find that a drug is giving you side effects, talk to your physician. Maintaining open communication with your medical team will ensure that you receive the treatment that you need.

Chapter 12

future directions in prostate treatment

What Happens in this Chapter

- Taking part in a clinical trial
- New advances in BPH
- New advances in prostate cancer treatment

Prostate therapy is always evolving and patients today can both benefit from advances that have already taken place and help spur on further improvements by taking part in clinical trials. Future technologies may include more targeted radiation treatment and sophisticated robotic techniques.

Clinical Trials and You

THE KEY TO ALL NEW MEDICAL ADVANCES IS CLINICAL RESEARCH—
research on real people. The purpose of clinical research trials is to
find out whether a particular medication, device, or technique is
both effective and safe. If you are eligible to take part in any of these
studies, you will be helping to test new treatments and playing a
direct role in providing new options for treating prostate disease.

Clinical trials may be sponsored by a pharmaceutical company,
biotechnology company, or a government agency, but all trials must
be officially approved by the hospital and independent ethics review
boards before a study can begin. In most trials, neither patients nor
researchers know until the end of the trial which patients are
receiving the treatment itself or a **placebo** (non-active treatment).
The advantage of this "double-blind" approach is that the results are
non-biased. The potential disadvantage for patients—aside from the
chance of finding out that the new therapy is ineffective—is that they
may find themselves in the placebo group and not actually receive the
new therapy.

If you have BPH, you may be asked to participate in a clinical trial
when you are first diagnosed, perhaps to test a new medication
designed to prevent surgery. If you have prostate cancer, you may be
offered the chance to test a new drug that fights prostate cancer
before surgery, or improves treatment afterward. Your physician will
determine whether you are eligible for a clinical trial and approach
you to take part; however, the decision is always yours. If you are not
interested, it will not affect the quality of your care in any way.

If you are interested in getting involved in a clinical research trial,
your best bet is to ask your physician. The Internet is another good
way to find out about clinical trials involving patients like you (e.g.,
www.clinicaltrials.gov).

New Advances in Benign Prostate Disease

The most promising new technique that provides an alternative to TURP is laser removal of the prostate gland. The procedure is similar to TURP in many respects, except that the obstructing prostate tissue is removed with a device called the Holmium laser. Although the technique still needs to be thoroughly tested and is not widely available, the results so far look good. It also appears to be easier on patients and reduces both hospital stay and recovery times.

New Advances in Radiation Therapy

Although external beam radiotherapy isn't new, combining it with chemotherapy is. Scientists are investigating the benefits of giving external radiation therapy to chemotherapy patients before and after their radiation treatment.

New Advances in Radical Prostatectomy

Laparoscopic techniques for radical prostatectomy are now being investigated around the world after French doctors reported success with this approach in the late 1990s. **Laparoscopic prostatectomy** involves making three or four tiny incisions instead of one large one and using thin telescopic instruments, guided by an image on a TV monitor, to remove the prostate gland. Laparoscopy can be done directly by the surgeon or with robotic arms that the surgeon controls—in the same room as the patient or even from a remote location.

Laparoscopic surgery in other areas of medicine has shown great benefits in terms of quicker recoveries and shorter hospital stays. Another advantage is that, as robotic technology improves, there is the potential for a surgeon to operate from a distant hospital—a plus for remote communities. However, it's still not clear whether laparoscopic approaches truly have advantages over the standard technique in prostate cancer, especially as the standard technique is so refined that small incisions and fast recovery are already the norm. There is concern that laparoscopy may not remove tumors as effectively as the standard technique, while providing only small advantages in terms of patient discomfort. Only time and further research will determine whether minimally invasive surgery is the way forward in the treatment of prostate disease.

Chemotherapy is also being investigated as an additional treatment for radical prostatectomy patients.

Chapter 13

who's who of hospital staff

What Happens in this Chapter

- Hospital staff you will meet
- A brief description of their roles

WHEN YOU GO INTO THE HOSPITAL, YOU WILL ENCOUNTER A LARGE number of staff. In general, they will be friendly and helpful. If you are dealing with them directly, they should introduce themselves and explain their roles to you.

However, it can be confusing that many of the hospital staff, from porters to doctors, wear a white coats or "scrubs" (loose pants and tops of different colors), making it hard to figure out who's who. Also, within the title of "doctor" or "nurse" are a number of different roles, making it difficult to understand what each of these people do. For example, you may see a **fellow**, a **resident**, or a **staff physician**. All are doctors, but have varying levels of knowledge, ability, and responsibility. Or, you may see a **ward nurse**, a **recovery room nurse**, or a **research nurse**. Again, all are qualified nurses, but each has a different role.

This chapter will give you a brief overview explaining who is who in the hospital and each person's role in your care.

[MORE DETAIL]

Medical Staff	Nursing Staff	Support Staff
Anesthesiologist	Community care access coordinator/homecare nurse	Blood technician
Fellow		Chaplain/pastor/priest
Medical student		Clerk
Oncologist	Nurse anesthetist (CRNA)	Dietitian
Pathologist	Nurse practitioner	ECG technician
Radiologist	Registered nurse	Patient care assistant/orderly/nurse's aid
Resident	Research nurse	Volunteer
Surgeon		

Anesthesiologist

A doctor who administers anesthesia to reduce or eliminate pain and put surgery patients to sleep. The anesthesiologist's job includes medically evaluating patients before surgery, consulting with the surgical team, providing pain control, support of life during surgery, making decisions about blood conservation and transfusions, supervising care after surgery, and discharging patients from the recovery unit or the intensive care unit.

Blood Technician

A person qualified to take blood from patients.

Certified Registered Nurse Anesthetist (CRNA)

A specially trained nurse who assists the anesthesiologist in caring for a patient while that patient is under anesthesia. A CRNA will also evaluate patients before surgery, care for them as they recover from anesthesia and carry out patient education.

Chaplain/Pastor/Priest/Rabbi

A person who is ordained to be a religious leader. He or she can provide counseling and prayer. The chaplain may be non-denominational.

Clerk

This is usually the first person you will meet when you arrive at the ward. He or she is responsible for answering the phone in the ward, but his or her role often extends beyond this, depending on experience level.

Community Care Access Co-ordinator/Homecare Nurse

In some hospitals, this nurse will work with your community and co-ordinate your care after you're discharged from the hospital.

Dietitian

This professional assists the health care team with recommendations regarding a patient's diet. A dietitian's advice is especially important for the team caring for people with diabetes or who have special food restrictions.

ECG Technician

A person who is specifically trained to perform ECGs on patients.

Fellow

A fully qualified doctor who has specialized in a particular area of medicine or surgery, usually with a few years of experience. Fellows can come from other countries to spend up to 3 years gaining additional experience.

Medical Student

A person who is enrolled in medical school and is being trained to become a medical doctor.

Nurse Practitioner

A registered nurse who has completed a master's degree in nursing. He or she performs advanced physical examinations and takes patients' medical histories. The nurse practitioner is also responsible for the coordination of patient care and patient education and works both independently and in collaboration with the health care team in making rounds, ordering diagnostic tests, interpreting the results, and deciding on treatment.

Oncologist

A physician who specializes in the diagnosis and treatment of cancer; individual oncologists usually specialize in just one type of cancer. You will mainly deal with oncologists interested in prostate cancer.

There are three types of oncologists you may encounter: a **surgical oncologist**, a **radiation oncologist**, and a **medical oncologist**. Your surgical oncologist will be a urologist with further credentials in the field of cancer surgery. A radiation oncologist deals with all types of radiation treatments for cancer. A medical oncologist specializes in the administration of drugs for the treatment of cancer, such as chemotherapy.

Pathologist

A doctor who specializes in examining and analyzing tissue samples under a microscope. This is the person who assigns tumors their Gleason score.

Patient Care Assistant/Orderly/Nurse's Aide

A trained member of the health care team who provides patient care under the supervision of a nurse. He or she may be the one to accompany you to tests or procedures.

Radiologist

A doctor who specializes in reading radiological tests, such as X-rays, ultrasounds, and CAT scans.

Registered Nurse

The nurse who is primarily responsible for your basic care and helps to coordinate, plan, and assess your needs throughout your surgical experience. He or she works closely with your surgeon. In bigger teaching centers, in particular, nurses may function in different capacities, such as a **recovery room (PACU) nurse**, **operating room nurse**, or a **nurse manager**.

Research Nurse

A nurse, usually with a university degree, who specializes in assisting and coordinating research. It is his or her job to approach patients for possible participation in research studies and coordinate their involvement. In some instances, the research nurse is also responsible for collecting blood samples for the studies and will see participants at follow-up appointments.

Resident

A physician who has completed medical school and is undergoing specialized training. He or she can specialize in a particular area, such as surgery or oncology (cancer care). If you are having your surgery at a university-affiliated hospital, you will encounter many residents. Although they are still in training, residents are certified physicians and are considered "front-line" workers. They take 24-hour call shifts and are just minutes away if an emergency arises. At teaching hospitals, in particular, they are vital to excellent patient care.

Surgeon

A doctor who specializes in performing surgery. Your urologist performs your surgery with the assistance of a resident or a private assistant and supervises your care before and after surgery.

Volunteer

A person who donates his or her time to the hospital. He or she may have one of a wide variety of roles.

Disclaimer: The above descriptions are intended as a general guide only. The roles of each type of staff member mentioned may differ slightly from hospital to hospital.

glossary

Adenocarcinoma The most common type of prostate cancer.

Analgesic Medication that relieves pain.

Anesthetic A drug used to block pain. Radical prostatectomy and TURP can be done under general anesthetic, which means you are completely asleep and will not feel any pain, or regional anesthetic, which means you will be numbed from the waist down, but will remain awake.

Antibiotic A medication for treating bacterial infections.

Anticoagulant A blood-thinning medication that decreases the chances of blood clots.

Antiemetic Medication to relieve nausea.

Autologous blood donation Storing your own blood before surgery to be used in the event that you need a blood transfusion.

Benign Non-cancerous, or non-malignant.

Benign prostatic hyperplasia (BPH) Non-cancerous growth of the prostate; occasionally called benign prostatic hypertrophy.

Biopsy A procedure to remove a sample of tissue and analyze it under a microscope in order to help make a diagnosis.

Bladder The muscular pouch-like organ that stores and excretes urine produced by the kidneys.

Bone scan A nuclear medicine test that is performed to see bones and assess bone health; it can detect abnormalities such as arthritis, fractures, and cancer.

Cancer Abnormal cells that grow uncontrollably.

Carcinoma Malignant tumor that originates in the lining or surface of an organ.

CAT scan *See* Computerized axial tomography.

Catheter A narrow tube that is inserted into a part of the body.

Clinical staging The doctor's estimate of the extent of the cancer.

Clinical trials Studies performed to evaluate the effectiveness of new or experimental treatments, or existing treatments for different types of patients.

149

Computerized axial tomography (CAT) scan Computer-generated cross-sectional images of the body.

Cystoscopy A procedure performed by a urologist using a scope inserted through the urethra to see inside the urethra, bladder, and prostate.

Detrusor muscle The muscle layer that surrounds the bladder and allows it to contract during urination.

Digital rectal exam (DRE) An examination of the prostate in which a lubricated gloved finger is inserted into the rectum and the prostate is felt through the rectum wall.

Ejaculation The release of semen from the penis during orgasm.

Epidural A small, thin tube placed in the spine through which medication can be given; used for anesthesia and pain management.

Erectile dysfunction A problem in achieving and maintaining an erection.

Frequency A frequent need to urinate.

Gleason grading system A scoring system for describing how aggressive prostate cancer is.

Hesitancy Difficulty in starting urine flow.

Hot spots Abnormalities on a bone scan, which may indicate arthritis, previous bone fractures, or tumors.

Impotence Inability to achieve or maintain an erection; the causes may be pathological or psychological.

Incision A cut made by the surgeon during surgery.

Incontinence Partial or total loss of urinary control.

Intramuscular (IM) Injected into the muscle.

Intravenous (IV) Injected into a vein.

Kegel exercises Pelvic muscle exercises used to help strengthen the muscles that control urination.

Laparoscopic radical prostatectomy Surgery to remove the prostate that is performed through small incisions, using small, telescope-like instruments.

Libido Sexual desire or "sex drive."

LUTS Lower urinary tract symptoms. A group of symptoms caused by urinary obstruction or an overactive bladder. *See also* Frequency, Hesitancy, Incontinence, Nocturia.

Lymph nodes Clusters of grape-shaped tissues found throughout the body (e.g., in the groin, neck, and underarms) that help defend the body against infections.

Magnetic resonance imaging (MRI) A test that uses magnetic and radio waves to produce detailed pictures of internal body structures.

Malignant Cancerous.

Margins The cut edge of tissue removed during surgery—a positive surgical margin means that cancer cells are visible at the outer edge of the removed tissue, indicating that cancer cells may remain in the body; a negative margin means there are no visible cancer cells, which may indicate that there are no cancer cells left behind in the body.

Metastasis Spread of cancer beyond where it originated; prostate cancer tends to spread to the lymph nodes and bones.

MRI *See* Magnetic resonance imaging.

Nocturia Frequent need to urinate during the night.

Oncologist A doctor who specializes in treating cancer.

Orgasm Sexual climax.

PACU *See* Patient anesthetic care unit.

Pathologist A doctor who specializes in analyzing tissue samples.

Patient anesthetic care unit (PACU) The "recovery room" in which you will recover following your surgery, before returning to the ward.

Pathological staging The evaluation of tissue removed during surgery.

Perineum The area between the scrotum and anus.

Perineal prostatectomy The surgical removal of the prostate through an incision in the perineum.

Peripheral intravenous line (PIV) A small tube that is placed in the vein to administer fluids and medication during and after surgery.

Peripheral zone The outer region of the prostate, where most prostate cancers are located.

Prognosis A prediction of how cancer will progress.

Prostate A walnut-sized gland located below the bladder that helps produce semen during ejaculation.

Prostate specific antigen (PSA) A protein produced by the prostate gland; high PSA levels could mean the presence of prostate cancer.

Prostatitis Inflammation and infection of the prostate.

Radical prostatectomy Complete surgical removal of the prostate.

Radiologist A doctor who specializes in reading and interpreting X-rays, CAT scans, and other radiological tests.

Retrograde ejaculation Occurs when semen flows up into the bladder during ejaculation due to bladder-neck damage; occurs frequently after trans-urethral resection of the prostate (TURP).

Scrotum The sack, containing the testicles, that hangs behind the penis.

Sedative A medication to relax you.

Semen Fluid released during orgasm that contains sperm and other fluids involved in ejaculation.

Seminal vesicles Small glands that excrete fluid into the semen during orgasm.

Sexual dysfunction The inability to get, or maintain, an erection.

Stage A measure of how far the cancer has spread.

Staples Used in closing an incision. May be used internally as well.

Stent A thin, flexible tube used to support body "tubes" such as arteries or the ureters.

Sutures Used in closing an incision; may be dissolvable or non-dissolvable.

Testicles Part of the male genitals, located within the scrotum behind the penis, that produce sperm and testosterone.

Testosterone The primary male sex hormone that is responsible for the development of male characteristics; may encourage the growth of prostate cancer.

Transition zone Innermost area of the prostate that surrounds the urethra as it exits the bladder.

Trans-rectal ultrasound An ultrasound of the prostate that uses a probe inserted through the rectum.

Transurethral resection of the prostate (TURP) Surgical removal of the tissue that is obstructing the urethra.

Tumor An abnormal lump of tissue.

TURP *See* Transurethral resection of the prostate.

Ultrasound A diagnostic test that uses sound waves to create an image of internal tissues.

Ureters Two small tubes that carry urine from the kidneys to the bladder.

Urethra The tube that allows urine and ejaculate to be excreted.

Urethral stricture Scarring or narrowing of the urethra.

Urinary retention Difficulty emptying the bladder due to blockage.

Urologist A surgeon who specializes in problems associated with the kidneys, ureters, bladder, prostate, urethra, and testicles.

Vas deferens Two small, muscular tubes that carry sperm into the urethra.

resources

Prostate and Cancer Information

American Urological Association
1120 North Charles Street
Baltimore, MD 21201
Tel: (410) 727-1100
Fax: (410) 223-4370
Patient information, the latest
research, and publications.
aua@auanet.org

"Well Connected" Health Features
Public Relations Department
Morehead Memorial Hospital,
117 E. Kings Highway,
Eden, North Carolina, 27288 USA
Tel: (336) 623-9711
Comprehensive articles on BPH and
prostate cancer.
http://www.morehead.org/feature.html

General Health Information

HealthFinder
A service of the U.S. Department of
Health and Human Services that con-
nects you to publications, non-profit
organizations, databases, Websites, and
support groups.
http://www.healthfinder.gov

WebMD
Reliable health information including
news, disease and drug information,
health television guide, and tips for
making a personal health plan and for
searching the medical library.
http://www.webmd.com

Stress and Relaxation Information

**The Transcendental Meditation
Program**
Find out the benefits of, and how and
where to learn, transcendental meditation.
http://www.tm.org

Meditation Society of America
Concepts and techniques of meditation
plus suggested reading.
http://www.meditationsociety.com

American Yoga Association
General information on yoga, how to
get started and how to choose a qualified yoga instructor.
http://www.americanyogaassociation.org

Nutrition and Fitness Information

American Dietetic Association
Daily tips and features about nutrition.
http://www.eatright.org

Information on Alternative Therapies

National Center for Complementary and Alternative Medicine
Tel: (301) 231-7537, ext 5
Fax: (301) 495-4957

An official source of information, including links to other sites, current research, and scientific information.
http://www.nccam.nih.gov

Alternative Medicine Digest
What's new in alternative medicine.
http://www.alternativemedicine.com

MEDLINE Plus
Information on herbal remedies.
http://www.nlm.nih.gov/medlineplus/herbalmedicine.html

Contact Information

Name of current family doctor:	Address:	Phone #:	Fax:	Email:
Hospitals:	Address:	Phone#:	Fax:	Email:
Name of your urologist:	Address:	Phone#:	Fax:	Email:

Medical Appointments

	Time	Address	Hospital
Pre-operative Dates			
Prostate Surgery Date	Time	Address	Hospital
Post-operative Date	Time	Address	Doctor
Annual Check-up Date	Time	Address	Doctor
PSA Date	Time	Address	Doctor

Current and Past Medications
(including complementary therapies and supplements)

Drug Name	Date Began Drug	Purpose of Drug	Dosage	Side Effects	Dosage Instructions

Symptoms

Symptom	Date	Time	Cause	Severity on scale of 1 to 10 (1=mild, 10=severe)	Duration

Questions for the Doctor

Taking Control of Your Life

Support Group and Counselor Contact Information

Address	Phone	Fax	Email

My Lifestyle Goals: Current Weight _____

index

References to figures: *3fig*;
references to tables: *119t*;
references to More Detail boxes in bold: **4**;
references to Key Point boxes in bold italic: ***5***;
references to Self-Help boxes in italic: *12*

5-alpha-reductase inhibitors, 31-32, 129-130, *136t*
acute urinary retention, 9, 29. *See also* urinary retention; voiding, problems with.
adenomas, 6
adrenergics, 29-30
alliums, 115
alpha blockers, 31-32, 129, *136t*
androgens, 40-41
anemia, 41, 58, 59, **60**, 61
anemia therapy, 131, *136t*
anesthetics, 70-71, *71*, 78. *See also* general anesthetic; regional anesthetic.
anesthesiologist, 54, 70-71, *71*
antiandrogens, 42, 130, *136t*
antibiotics, 131, *136t*
anticholinergic drugs, 83, 98-99, 134
anticoagulants, *136t*
anti-embolic stockings 65, **67**
anti-emetics, 134, *137t*
anti-inflammatory drugs, ***54***
artificial urinary sphincter, 99-100
atypical small acinar cell proliferation (ASAP), 21
AUA symptom score, 14, **15**

benign prostatic hyperplasia (BPH), 1, 5, 6-9, *7fig*; causes of, **10**; contra-indicated medications for, 29-31; diagnosis of, 14, **15**; diet and, 113; future trends in treatment of, 141; medications for, 31-32, *35t*, 129-130, *136t*; PSA test and, **18**; quality of life and, 8, 29-32; symptoms of, **6**, 8-9, 29-32; treatment options for, 1-2, 28-35, *30*, **34**, *35t*
biopsy, 19-22, *20*, *22*
bladder neck stricture, 45
bladder spasm, 134, *137t*
bladder stones, 8-9, 16
blood conservation strategies, 59-61
blood donation (autologous), 59-60
blood transfusions, 44, 57-61, **60**
bone scan, 27
bowel prep, 57
BPH. *See* benign prostatic hyperplasia.
brachytherapy, 37-40, ***39***
breathing exercises, 84
CAT scan, 24, 26
catheter. *See* urinary catheter.
catheter care, 89-91, *90*
chemotherapy, 141, 142

clinical trials, 140
complementary therapies, 108-116, *114*, 116
computerized axial tomography. *See* CAT scan.
conformal radiotherapy, 39
consent, 55-56, **56**
continuous bladder irrigation, 73, **81**
coughing, 84
cystoscopy, 16
deep vein thrombosis, **67**, 85
diet, 113-116, **113**
digital rectal exam (DRE), 16-17
dihydrotestosterone (DHT), **10**, 129-130
diuretics, 30-31
diverticulae, 32
DRE. *See* digital rectal exam.
driving, 91
drug therapy, for BPH, 31-32, *35t*; for prostate cancer, 40-42. *See also* medications.
emotions, post-surgery, 106-108; pre-surgery, 49-52, 62, 65
erectile dysfunction, 116-117, *117*; following radical prostatectomy, 45, 100-103, *101*, 126; following TURP, 33-34, 95; medications for, 92, 102-103, *103*, 135, *137t*
erythropoietin, 59, 131, *136t*
estrogen, **10**
exercise. *See* physical activity.
external beam radiotherapy, 37-39, 141
flying, 92
Foley catheter, 79-81, *80fig*, **81**
follow-up visits, 93
frequency, *6*, 8, **15**
future trends, 139-142
general anesthetic, 66, 70, 71, 132-133, *132*, *137t*
Gleason score, 22-24, **23**

guided imagery, 111
hematuria, **6**, 9
hemolytic reactions, 58
high-intensity ultrasound, 34
Holmium laser, 141
hormone treatment, 40-42, *46t*, 124, *136t*
hospital admission, 64-65
hospital checklists, 63, 86
hospital discharge, 85-86
hospital staff, 143-148
incontinence, 45, 47; following radical prostatectomy, 96-100, **99**, 126; following TURP, 94
infection, control of, 88-91
intensity modulated radiotherapy (IMRT), 39
intraurethral stents, 34
Jackson-Pratt drain, 76
Kegel exercises, 94, 97, *98*
laparascopic prostatectomy, 141-142
laparoscopy, 66, **75**, 141-142
laxatives, 134
LHRH agonists. *See* luteinizing hormone-releasing hormone agonists.
lower urinary tract symptoms, 6-9, 14-16, **15**, 29-32, *34*; measuring improvement of, 120-121
luteinizing hormone-releasing hormone (LHRH) agonists, 41-42, 130, *136t*
LUTS. *See* lower urinary tract symptoms.
lycopenes, 115
magnetic resonance imaging. *See* MRI.
male sling procedure, 99
malignant hyperthermia, 54
massage, 111
medications, 128-138; as treatment for BPH, 31-32, *35t*, 129-130; as treatment for prostate cancer, 130;

before surgery, 131; contra-
indicated before biopsies, **20**;
contra-indicated before surgery, **54**;
contra-indicated for BPH, 29-31;
for bladder spasm, 133, 134, *137t*;
for erectile dysfunction, 92, 102-
103, **103**, 134-135, *137t*; for
incontinence, 98-99, 134-135,
137t; hormone, 40-42, *46t*, 124,
136t; pain relief, 83, **83**, 133, *137t*;
possible side effects of, **18**, 130, 135,
136t-137t; post-surgery, 133-135
meditation, 110
metastases, 24
micro-metastasis, 125
minimally invasive treatments, 34, 141-142
MRI, 26-27
nerve-sparing, **44**, 45, 101, 126
nocturia, 8
pain management, 82-84, **83**, *137t*
pathology report, 121-122, *123fig*
patient-controlled analgesia, 83-84, **83**
penile implant surgery, 103
perineal radical prostatectomy, **75**
peripheral zone, 5, *7fig*
phosphodiesterase-5 (PDE5) inhibitors,
102, **103**, *137t*
physical activity, 85, 91, **92**, 112, **112**
pis en deux, 8
polyphenols, 115
post-anesthesia recovery unit (PACU),
78, **78**
pre-admission clinic, 53-54
pre-admission procedures, 48-64
pre-donating blood. *See* autologous blood
donation.
pre-surgery, 62-68, 131
priapism, 103
prostaglandins, 102-103, *137t*
prostate cancer, 1-2, 5, 9-12; adjuvant

treatment of, 124; diagnosis of, 11-
12, 16-27, **23**; diet and, 114-116;
early detection of, 9-12; measuring
treatment of, 121-126; medications
for, 40-42, 130; symptoms of, *11fig*,
11-12; treatment options for, 1, 9-11,
36-47, **38**, *46t*
prostate disease, 1-12; diagnosis of, 13-27;
future trends in treatment of, 139-
142; treatment options for, 1, 28-47
prostate enlargement, 2, 6-9, *7fig*, **10**
prostate gland, anatomy of, 1, 3-6, *3fig*,
5fig, *7fig*; enlargement of, 2, 6-9, *7fig*,
10; laser removal of, 141; re-growth
of following surgery, 96; removal of,
43; urethra and, 4-6, *5fig*. *See also*
radical prostatectomy; transurethral
resection of the prostate.
prostate specific antigen (PSA) test, 17-
19, **18**, 24 ; post-surgery, 124-125,
125
prostatectomy. *See* radical prostatectomy.
prostatic intraepithelial neoplasia (PIN), 21
prostatitis, 2, **18**
PSA test. *See* prostate specific antigen test.
PSA velocity, **18**
quality of life, BPH and, 8; prostate
cancer and, 125-126
questions to ask, 50, *51*
radiation therapy, 9-11, 37-40; as adjuvant
treatment, 124, **124**; future trends in,
141; vs. surgery, **38**, *46t*
radical prostatectomy, advantages of,
43; anesthesia for, 66, 70, 71, 132-
133, *137t*; as treatment option, 1, 42-
47, **43**, *46t*; blood transfusions and,
57-61; bowel prep, 57; consent for,
55-56, **56**; erectile dysfunction
following, 100-103, 126; follow-up
visits for, 93; future trends in, 141-

142; incontinence following, 96-100, **99**; possible risks or side effects of, 44-47, 96-104; pre-surgery, 48-68; procedure, 70-71, 74fig, 74-76; quality of life following, 125-126; recovery from, 77-118; sex following, 92, 100-103, *101*, *103*; variations on, **75**; work, time off from, 52, 92

radiotherapy. *See* radiation therapy.

recovery, at home, 87-93; in hospital, 77-86

rectal injury, 103

rectoscope, 72-73, 72fig

regional anesthetic, 70-71, *132*, 133

relaxation techniques, 110-111

reminiscence therapy, 111

repeat biopsies, 21

reproductive system, prostate and, *3fig*, 4-6, *5fig*

results, of TURP, 119-121; of radical prostatectomy, 119, 121-126

retrograde ejaculation, 34, 95-96

risks of radical prostatectomy, 44-47

saturation biopsy, 21

saw palmetto, 31, 113

sedatives, 131

self-care, 22, 49-52; *98*, 105-118

self-catheterization, 33, 94

semen, 4, *5fig*

sex, 92, 95-96, 100-103, 116-117

side effects, possible, following radical prostatectomy, 96-104; following TURP, 94-96; of medications, 130, 135, *136t-137t*

sleep, 113

smooth muscle relaxants. *See* anticholinergic drugs.

sound therapy, 111

soy, 115

stool softeners, 134, *137t*

stress incontinence, 47, 94

stress management, 109-113

support groups, *50*, 107-108

surgical margins, 122-124, *123fig*

testosterone, **10**, 40-42

tests and measurements, for BPH, 13-14, **15**; for lower urinary tract symptoms, 13-16, **15**; for prostate cancer, 11, 16-27, **23**; for success of radical prostatectomy, 121-126; for success of TURP, 120, 121; pre-admission, 53

TNM staging system, 24

transition zone, 5, 6, *7fig*

transrectal ultrasound-guided biopsy, 19-20

transurethral balloon dilation, 34

transurethral electrovaporization, 34

transurethral hyperthermia, 34

transurethral microwave thermotherapy (TUMT), 34

transurethral needle ablation (TUNA), 34

transurethral resection of the prostate (TURP), advantages of, 32-33, *35t*; anesthesia for, 66, 132-133, *132*, *137t*; consent for, 55-56, **56**; erectile dysfunction following, 95, 100-103; follow-up visits for, 93; medications during, 132-133; possible risks and side effects of, 33-34, *35t*, 94-96; pre-surgery, 48-56, 62-68; procedure, 69-73, *72fig*; recovery from, 77-118; results of, 119-121; sex following, 92, 95; work, time off from, 52, 92

treatment options, for BPH, 1-2, 28-35, *30*, **34**, *35t*; for erectile dysfunction, 100-103; for incontinence, 94, 97-100, **99**; for prostate cancer, 1, 9-11, 36-47, **38**, *46t*, 124; for prostatitis, 2; future trends in, 139-142

tubes, 73, 79-82, *80fig*, **81**

tumors, 9-11, *11fig*, 22-27. *See also* prostate cancer.

TURP. *See* transurethral resection of the prostate.

ultrasound, abdominal, 15-16; high-intensity, 34; transrectal, 19-20

uretal injury, 104

urethral meatus, 89-90

urethral stricture, 16

urethra-prostate connection, 4-6, *5fig*

urge incontinence, 94, 97, 98-99

urgency, *6*

urinary catheter, 9, 73, *74fig*, 75, 79-81, *80fig*, **81**, 85; care of, 89-91, *90*; intermittent self-catheterization, 33, 94; removal of, 93, *93*, 120

urinary leakage, *6*, 96-97, 121, 126

urinary retention, *6*, 9, 29-32, 33, 93; following radical prostatectomy, 96; following TURP, 94

urinary system, 3-4, *3fig*

urinary tract infections. *See* lower urinary tract symptoms.

urination. *See* voiding.

urine collection bag, 79-81, *80fig*, **81**, 89, 90

urine crystals, 9

uroflow test, 14, 121

vacuum erection device (VED), 102

visual internal urethotomy, 96

visualization, 111

vitamin E, *54*, 114

vitamins and supplements, 114-116, *114*; to avoid, 115-116

voiding trial, 120

voiding, problems with, 6-9, *6*, *7fig*, **15**, 29-32; following radical prostatectomy, 96; following TURP, 94. *See also* incontinence; lower urinary tract symptoms; urinary retention.

watchful waiting, 9-11, 29-31, *35t*, **36**, 36-37, *46t*

weight management, 112

work, time off from, 52, 92

wound care, 88-89, *88*